Elizabeth
Devine

Appearances

A Complete
Guide to
Cosmetic
Surgery

PIATKUS

© 1982 Elizàbeth Devine

First published in Great Britain in 1982
by Judy Piatkus (Publishers) Limited
of Loughton, Essex

British Library Cataloguing in Publication Data

Devine, Elizabeth
  Appearances: a complete guide to cosmetic surgery.
  1. Surgery, Plastic
  I. Title
  617'.95   RD119

ISBN 0-86188-178-8

Typeset by V & M Graphics Ltd, Aylesbury, Bucks
Printed and bound by Mansell (Bookbinders) Witham, Essex. .

To Connie and Jim,
who have given years of friendship,

to George,
who changed my life,

and to Patrick,
who has been a lesson in generosity

Contents

Acknowledgements

Except for Marti Caine and Tony Hiller, I have used fictitious names for all persons quoted or referred to in this book who have had plastic surgery. In some cases I have changed place names as well.

I thank the many persons—British and American, patients, surgeons, and others—who have given me invaluable help in preparing this book: Dr William Adams, Ms Terry Bagley, Ms Liz Barrett, Ms Carol Blanks, Ms Marti Caine, Ms Maria Campbell, Mr Neil Cathcart, Ms Constance Clark, Dr John Constable, Dr Charles Darley, Mr Peter Davis, Ms Eileen Devine, Dr Matthias Donelan, Ms Muriel Emmanuel, Dr Sidney Feuerstein, Dr O. S. Frank, Dr Raghu Gaind, Mr Leslie Gardiner, Dr Patrick Guinan, Harrods Trichology Department administrators and personnel, Dr Dana Heikes, Mr Tony Hiller, Dr Fred H. Horne, Dr A. G. Huff, Dr Mary Israel, Mr Percy Jayes, Ms Gail Katz, Dr Fred Kingsley, Ms Alix Kirsta, Ms Maureen Lambert, Dr Ronald Lande, Mr Philip Lebon, Dr Mark Lewis, Dr Elmer Mitchell, Jr, Mr Alan Moore, Dr Fred A. Pezzulli, Dr Thomas Planek, Ms Marie Pocknell, Mr Peter Pocknell, Mr Leonard Pountney, Dr Leon Remis, Ms R. Roberts, Ms Donnalee Rubin, Mr Patrick Ryan, Mr R. P. G. Sandon, Dr Sheldon Sevinor, Ms June Sinclair, Ms Carol Snell, Dr Richard Boies Stark, Tao Clinic administrators and personnel, Dr Jerry Tuttle, Mr William Ursell, Mr Patrick Whitfield, Mr Charles Whittaker, Mr Derek Wilson, and Ms Sally Wilson.

I also am most grateful to the many persons—both patients and surgeons—who shared their time, their experiences, and their expertise with me but who wish to remain anonymous.

Finally, I thank Ms Julie Garriott, the most astute and supportive editor a writer could wish for.

ELIZABETH DEVINE

Prologue

1 The Decision

It is only shallow people who do not judge by appearances.—Oscar Wilde

For many people, holding the mirror up to nature in a frank appraisal of one's appearance isn't an altogether pleasant experience.

Mother Nature has been very generous with the Diana Riggs and the Roger Moores, but most of us have been dealt a mistake or two: a nose that doesn't complement our other facial features, too-prominent ears, a flat chest ...

And we all eventually fall victim to another of Nature's little tricks: ageing. At a certain point in our lives, what used to be firm starts sagging.

Which limitations or idiosyncrasies in our physical appearance can we live with more or less comfortably? Which may we feel strongly enough about to want to change? Such feelings are a very personal matter. One person may live contentedly, even proudly, with a nose that looks like an eagle's beak; another with a similarly imposing proboscis may refuse to be photographed out of self-consciousness.

People who want to change a physical feature are turning in increasing numbers to cosmetic surgery, or aesthetic surgery, as it is sometimes called.

'Cosmetic surgery' is a term that, to most of us, sounds self-contradictory. *Surgery* is a word we usually avoid using unless a serious health problem is involved; *cosmetic* suggests a tube of lip gloss from the local chemist—something simple to get and easy to use that will enhance our looks temporarily and superficially.

Cosmetic surgery *is* different from other surgery—even from other plastic surgery. Most people who have surgery are told by a doctor that an operation is necessary or advisable to maintain or restore good health. Certainly we have been conditioned to avoid surgery, not to seek it out. But in the case of cosmetic surgery, the patient makes the diagnosis that something is wrong and asks for an operation, to alter a nose, perhaps, or to enlarge breasts or transplant hair.

The best way to understand cosmetic surgery is to see it in relation to the other branch of plastic surgery, reconstructive surgery. Although both types of plastic surgery use the same techniques, they have different aims. A London doctor says, 'Reconstructive plastic surgery attempts to make the body part in question—a nose, a breast, a burned area—normal. With cosmetic surgery, the anatomical body part is normal, but the aim is to increase the acceptability of the appearance of that feature—in other words, to improve on the normal.'

Some cosmetic surgery is not exclusively cosmetic: both cosmetic dentistry and jaw surgery often correct a faulty bite; breast reduction is often performed mainly to relieve discomfort and difficulties in posture. But we may call such operations cosmetic because they often do dramatically improve one's appearance.

Forty-five-year-old Caroline Talmadge went to a plastic surgeon six weeks after her husband of twenty-five years died. Reading a woman's magazine, she had come across an article on cosmetic surgery and decided it might be easier to meet the world alone if she had a face lift.

Sandra Christopher had saved for three years with the idea of having a long holiday on the Continent *or* a breast augmentation operation. She decided to have the operation, 'because I've always been self-conscious about not having breasts. I'd just like to be able to get clothes that fit me—top and bottom—and I know I'd feel better if I wasn't always wondering whether my padded bra was slipping.'

Karen MacCleary came to the surgeon with her mother, Patricia. Karen was seventeen, with a very prominent nose. Patricia said, 'That nose runs in our family, but I want to give Karen a new nose for her birthday present.' Karen was agreeable, saying she didn't mind one way or the other.

Fred Lenox, a forty-seven-year-old salesman, learned that his company had just been bought by a larger firm. Instead of buying a new car, as he'd planned, he decided to use the money to have the bags under his eyes removed so that he'd look younger when the new management team took over.

Of these four applicants for cosmetic surgery, only Sandra Christopher is sure to be accepted, with Fred Lenox a close second. Both Caroline Talmadge and Karen MacCleary would be rejected by a responsible surgeon.

The surgeon would probably advise Caroline to return in six months if she still wanted the operation. It's not a good idea to have elective surgery if you're in the midst of a crisis—be it a divorce, the loss of a job, or the death of a spouse. Says a London psychiatrist, 'You should have such surgery when your feelings about yourself are basically good, not when you're under any particular duress.'

Karen MacCleary would also be turned down, because she is consenting to surgery to please not herself, but someone else.

The psychiatrist describes the differences in motives for cosmetic surgery: 'Motivation is absolutely crucial to whether surgery should be performed. There are two kinds of motivation: external and internal. "External" is related to things such as pressures from other people—from mother, from father, from husband—who think you ought to change. Or you may have a feeling that others will treat you differently after you've had the surgery. These are relative indications that the surgery shouldn't be done. If the pressure comes from within—you believe that you could look better, or you see the change as leading to an increase in self-confidence and your ability to deal with people—that is, on the whole, a favourable motivation.'

Fred Lenox would be questioned closely by the plastic surgeon, because surgeons do not want to operate on people who have unrealistic expectations about the results of cosmetic surgery. If Fred would rely on the surgery to save a job in jeopardy or win him a promotion, the surgeon will probably turn him down. If he mainly wants to look younger and more rested and thinks he'll feel happier about himself, he'll be a good risk for the procedure.

Sandra Christopher is a good candidate precisely because her attitude toward the results of the surgery *is* realistic. She expects to be able to wear the kinds of clothes she likes and to feel better about herself.

The best possible motive for cosmetic surgery is Sandra's—normal human vanity. It's best to leave other people's views of you out of the decision about having the surgery, if only because most people won't notice you've had something done. Astonishing though it may be, doctors and patients agree that people who know you will generally comment afterwards that you look good or that you look rested, but they really don't see that you have had a face lift or a nose job.

Alix Kirsta, health and beauty editor of *Woman's Own*, comments, 'In England, vanity is a dirty word. But it's the best motive. You look in the mirror and don't quite like what you see and want to have it improved. The bad motives are things like a woman saying, "My husband is having an affair with his secretary, and I know it's because my bust isn't big enough."'

For some people, the motive behind cosmetic surgery is primarily economic. Christine MacKay, a forty-two-year-old actress, decided to have a face lift 'to give myself a few more years before I started playing Shelley Winters parts.' And a rock star, thirty-four, came to a plastic surgeon and said, 'I can't very well keep playing to teenybopper audiences with these bags under my eyes, can I?'

The economic motive doesn't apply only to actors, models, and rock stars. In an interview with a plastic surgeon, Fred Lenox said he wanted the surgery as an economic investment in himself, because he felt a rested, more youthful image would build his confidence as a salesman.

If you're satisfied that your reason for wanting to have cosmetic surgery is simply a desire to look better, you're ready to face some other questions: Shall I talk it over with anyone? How do I find a plastic surgeon? What happens at the consultation?

2 Shall I Tell the World?

There are some things which men confess with ease, and others with difficulty.—Epictetus

People considering cosmetic surgery often have a hard time deciding whether to keep it a secret or to tell everyone in town. At least one woman who had breast augmentation didn't even tell her husband! She said she had to go into hospital because of a whiplash injury she'd suffered in a car accident, and she explained the change in her breasts by saying she was on a new birth control pill. (Either her husband is extremely gullible or he is a saint who knew what had happened and accepted that his wife couldn't discuss the subject with him.)

Adriana Clark's decision to have her nose altered was shared with her family and a small circle of friends, both male and female. For the most part, the women were very supportive and the men were indifferent or hostile. The most common pattern among women who have cosmetic surgery seems to be to tell their husband and one or two close female friends.

Not telling your spouse is very risky, says a London psychiatrist, because her or his feelings about the surgery can have a profound effect on your marriage. 'To go and have something done and not tell your spouse could be disastrous. It's inviting trouble.

'Sometimes I see couples when the wife wants cosmetic surgery and the husband doesn't want her to have it. In those cases I'm concerned about the relationship between them. Is this worry about a part of the body a reflection of a problem in their relationship?

'I would never attempt to change either one's mind. If there is a difference of perception between the two, I would advise against the operation until it's been resolved.

'A husband is often surprised about a wife's desire for cosmetic surgery and says he never noticed the problem. But, as is quite commonly the case, he may have teased her about her nose. She's had this condition and coped with it, and then under the impact of teasing from her husband, which is usually not intended to be unkind, the whole adolescent horror has been reactivated. Once he knows that, and she knows that he knows that, he may say, "Look, doctor, I think you ought to do it." Then, fine. If there isn't agreement, though, then I wouldn't recommend surgery.'

Understandably, a spouse may be sceptical about the surgery and its results. Sometimes the expense is an issue. Often it's a fear that the desire to change your appearance is a desire to become more attractive to the opposite sex; that it is a reflection of negative feelings about the marriage. A dermatologist says, 'If my partner were to feel that she wanted a face lift, I would think there was something wrong with our relationship, because that's something I shouldn't make her feel uncomfortable about and which she shouldn't feel uncomfortable about. If we can't go on enjoying our social lives and our family lives with a slightly more wrinkled skin than we might desire, it's very sad.'

The dermatologist has voiced fallacies often held by spouses of people who want cosmetic surgery. His wife would not have to be dissatisfied with their relationship to want a face lift for herself. Nor is the responsibility necessarily his if she is displeased with her appearance. She simply may feel that she doesn't look good, and looking good and feeling good very often go together. Oddly, a man who can understand why his wife would want to spend two thousand pounds on a fur coat sometimes cannot understand why she would want to spend less than half that on having her nose changed or her face lifted.

19

When James Lewis told his wife he wanted a hair transplant, she resisted the idea at first and assured him that she loved him with or without hair. When she realised that the transplant was important to him, she agreed that they would give up a holiday and a new car so that he could have it. She was so impressed with the results that she is now thinking of having her nose done.

Each marriage is different, so the decision of how and when to tell your spouse is a very personal one. Paulette Lynch made all the arrangements for her nose surgery and didn't tell her husband until the day before; there seems to have been no permanent damage to the marriage. Adriana Clark confided in her husband long before an opportunity arose to have nose surgery for much less than the usual cost. He didn't understand then why she wanted the surgery, and, though he cooperated in the process, he's still not entirely sure why she went to all the bother. But he admits her 'new' nose is much more attractive.

If you're satisfied that your motives are sound and your spouse cooperative, or at least neutral, you're ready to embark on the search for a cosmetic surgeon.

3 Finding a Surgeon

'Tis not too late to seek a newer world.—Alfred, Lord Tennyson

Finding a competent surgeon for a face lift should be no more difficult than finding someone to take out your gall bladder. But that isn't the case—thanks partly to the British medical establishment and partly to the jungle of commercial clinics that has sprung up since the mid-1970s.

There are some eighty consultant plastic surgeons in Great Britain, concentrated at hospitals with plastic surgery units. There are three in the London area: Mount Vernon Hospital in London, Queen Mary's Hospital in Roehampton, and Queen Victoria Hospital in East Grinstead, Sussex (where pioneering work in modern plastic surgery was done by Sir Archibald McIndoe). Other plastic surgery units are spread around the United Kingdom: in Billericay (Essex), Stoke Mandeville (Buckinghamshire), Salisbury, Leicester, Nottingham, Bristol, Chepstow, Leeds, Bradford, Liverpool, Manchester, Newcastle, Glasgow, Edinburgh, Aberdeen, and Belfast. These are plastic surgery units at National Health Service hospitals and should not be confused with private hospitals or commercial clinics.

There are three major problems in finding a competent and reliable plastic surgeon: the vagueness of medical standards, the aggressiveness of inferior commercial clinics, and, to a lesser extent, the reluctance of some general practitioners to refer patients to plastic surgeons.

21

First, in Britain *you don't have to be formally medically qualified to operate on someone.* According to a consultant plastic surgeon, 'The regulations regarding qualifications are fairly vague. It is not essential to be medically qualified to operate on people as long as you don't misrepresent yourself to be a doctor.

'If you're not a doctor and you purport to be able to do an operation and in fact you can't do it, you can be sued for negligence. Whether you're formally qualified or not, you do have an obligation to competence. You promise competence by saying you're going to do the operation. But, competent or not, you're still legally entitled to perform the surgery. A policeman couldn't stop you from performing an appendectomy or a face lift.'

This problem can manifest itself in two ways. Because anyone can legally perform surgery, some unqualified persons represent themselves as surgeons. A London doctor showed me a letter that had been passed on to him. It came from Scotland and was signed by Mr X, 'Surgeon and Practitioner'. Said the doctor, 'He's no more a surgeon than you are, but nothing can be done to stop him. The British Medical Association was approached, but they said that they had no jurisdiction.'

Another version of the qualification problem sometimes surfaces with a commercial clinic. Their advertisements may say, 'All surgery done under a surgeon's supervision' (or words to that effect). This may mean that there is a surgeon in the adjacent operating theatre, or merely that there is one somewhere in the building should something go wrong, while the actual surgery is being done by a physician without surgical training, or by a nurse.

Some procedures that pose little danger of complication (such as punch-graft hair transplants and electrolysis) can be done safely and effectively at clinics. However, just as with more complex cosmetic surgery, you should learn the background of the person who will perform the operation and the number of times he or she has performed it recently.

The second difficulty in finding a reliable plastic surgeon arises out of a rule that started with an honourable intention. There is a long tradition that those associated with the medical profession do not advertise. The rule was intended to protect patients, but instead makes it very difficult for some people to get medical services they would like to have, because of the very broad interpretation of the term 'advertising' by the General Medical Council.

You will notice that no physicians or surgeons are quoted by name in this book; they are identified as 'a consultant plastic surgeon', 'a psychiatrist', and so forth. Physicians and surgeons would not agree to interviews until they were assured and reassured that they would not be identified by name in the book, because such mention might be construed as advertising by the General Medical Council.

A few years ago, however, it became clear that clinics offering services such as family planning and vasectomies needed to advertise in order to get their messages to the public. The advertising rule was relaxed so that such clinics could advertise while still retaining the services of physicians and surgeons. However, the physicians and surgeons could not be mentioned by name in the advertisements.

Through this loophole crept many cosmetic surgery clinics and cosmetic surgery referral services, most of which seek clients by advertising in women's magazines and daily newspapers. Doctors work for all of them, but their names are not given in the advertisements.

Here's how many of these clinics operate. Mr A, a former hairdresser (several clinic owners are from the beauty field), who now calls himself a 'clinical consultant' or a 'surgical administrator', puts an advertisement in a women's magazine or a daily paper with an address and/or phone number where he can be reached for a referral. Mrs X, who would like to have cosmetic surgery, calls him. She is told to see Dr B, a general practitioner, who will give her a letter of referral to a cosmetic surgeon. She makes an appointment with Dr B, who refers her to a cosmetic surgeon, Mr C, at a nearby clinic.

In fact, Mr A, Dr B, and Mr C are in league with one

another and are splitting the fee that Mrs X pays. They may even be partners in the ownership of the clinic.

Legally, Mr A can advertise because he is a 'lay person', someone not connected with the medical profession. As a GP, Dr B supposedly has the best interests of the patient at heart and will refer her to a cosmetic surgeon skilled in the particular surgery she wants. In fact, he refers all patients to Mr C.

Says a London plastic surgeon, 'Some referral services pay lip service to the idea that the specialist should receive patients from a GP. They have *one* doctor, to whom *all* patients are referred. The usual GP would know that Smith rather than Jones would be the best surgeon for a certain operation.'

Two women who operate a cosmetic surgery referral service run an advertisement saying that they offer 'referrals to cosmetic *surgeons* [italics mine] in strictest confidence.' When asked how many cosmetic surgeons they have on their files to whom they refer patients, they say that they use just one. People who call them and confide their wish to have plastic surgery do not get an honest referral, much less a well-informed one.

Another surgeon describes his objections to this commercial referral process. 'They'll promise you the moon. What upsets me is that a lot of people are simple—in the nice sense of the word. They're honest, and they think that because they're paying a lot of money, what they're going to have is the best. Their expectations are quite large about the surgery. If things don't go right for them, they feel slightly ashamed that they were inveigled into spending this money to have something done. A good surgeon would have told them that the results couldn't come up to expectations he knew to be unrealistic.

'Then people are usually embarrassed to complain about it. Most just write it off as a bad financial experience, and I think they're being exploited.'

There are still other reasons against being operated on at a commercial clinic.

A surgeon appointed to the staff of a hospital has been judged for that appointment by other physicians and

24

surgeons; a surgeon hired by a commercial clinic is usually evaluated by a manager who is a business person and often has, at best, an educated layman's knowledge of medicine and surgery. Furthermore, the 'surgeon' working at a clinic may have no experience in surgery and no training in plastic surgery. What frequently counts most at clinics is how rapidly a surgeon can work. A clinic operator said that he had recently fired two surgeons who were Fellows of the Royal College of Surgeons: they weren't fast enough.

The patient pays a price, other than in pounds sterling, when being operated on at one of the commercial clinics. According to a plastic surgeon, 'These surgeons are on the fringes of the medical profession and often are unaware of important advances in the profession. They are removed from the standards that a hospital sets and from the day-to-day peer review as well as the intellectual stimulation of colleagues.'

Another plastic surgeon summarises his objections to the commercial clinics: 'The surgeon working at a clinic finds himself an employee of the clinic. Most other surgeons find it difficult to be convinced that he has an entirely free hand.

'At the clinic, by the time the patient sees the person who will do the surgery, he or she has paid a deposit and made a commitment to the surgery. The pressure is on the surgeon to perform the operation unless there is an overriding reason not to. The surgeon has the theoretical freedom to say no, but he probably cannot exercise that freedom very often.

'A physician or surgeon offers himself on his reputation. He is known through hospital standing, publications, etc. Qualified colleagues judge whether he deserves having patients sent to him. The clinics, however, are free to obtain the services of whatever medical personnel they can persuade to come to them. Sometimes the patient won't know the doctor's name until after the operation. He need not have passed any kind of acceptability test by a peer tribunal, as is the case for a hospital post. A surgeon at a clinic might be good—but it's just luck.

25

'Furthermore, conditions are not up to hospital standards. Often the air in the operating theatre isn't filtered, it's not air-conditioned, and the apparatus is inadequate.'

John Bealford, who had surgery at a clinic, reports they would not tell him the name of his surgeon until the morning of the operation. He was told that it was illegal to divulge the surgeon's name because the surgeon would be guilty of advertising. Bealford was surprised when he learned that the clinic's statement was untrue. When pressed, one clinic admitted that they wouldn't tell the name of the surgeon until the patient has put down a deposit on the operation: 'If we told who the surgeon was, the patient could simply contact him privately and have the work done without coming to our clinic.'

Yet another plastic surgeon says, 'The vast bulk of the medical profession has earned the trust that people put in them, and the commercial clinics cash in on that. Reputable plastic surgeons are distressed by injury to innocent people, by the besmirchment of our reputation, and by abuse of the trust the community holds us in.'

A standard practice at commercial clinics is for the patient to be admitted, operated on, and then sent home very soon—usually within hours—after the surgery is completed. This limits the time when trained medical staff are around for the crucial aftercare following an operation. A plastic surgeon explains, 'There can be bleeding, or there can be infection. The operation may have gone nicely, but inadequate or negligent aftercare can make the whole procedure a shambles. Medical staff will notice problems at an early stage, when the patient might not. One doesn't like to think about the infections that have made it necessary to perform surgery on a nose or a breast a second time. Some of those infections might well have been prevented with more attentive aftercare.'

Alix Kirsta has strong feelings about commercial cosmetic surgery clinics: 'All the clinics have to do to stay open is to get a licence and show that they're safe in case of fire. There is often no proper consultation with the patient. Frequently, they don't even do blood tests or take medical histories. And you can end up on the table without seeing the surgeon.

'Why do women allow a surgeon they've never seen to operate on them? Probably because they're ill-informed and scared. A woman is frightened when faced by a surgeon or doctor and usually thinks the surgeon's word is gospel. Medicine is a male-oriented profession, the last bastion of male chauvinism: I am the doctor. I am the autocrat.

'Ordinary people know cosmetic surgery is available, but they don't know whom to approach, so they go to those who advertise. Cosmetic surgery in clinics is overpriced and often botched. And women, mainly, are the victims. People are demanding access to cosmetic surgery, but they are not demanding quality. They end up having access to the wrong person.

'The medical profession must be educated, because they are helping to throw people into the arms of these clinics. Ten years ago, only the élite had this work done, so they knew they were being operated on by the best people. Now the charlatans have crept in, and people are getting access to really bad surgery.'

Kirsta's conclusions are reinforced by a surgeon who says, 'Just by the law of averages, it stands to reason that some of the surgery done at clinics will be fine. But patients are taking a terrible risk of being butchered.'

The Los Angeles *Times* reported the case of a woman who was operated on by a man who called himself a plastic surgeon, though his training was limited to ear, nose, and throat. He performed the operation in his office operating theatre, an environment similar to that found in some British clinics.

The case involved the death of Kim Plock, a woman on whom Dr Small was performing a breast-reduction operation in November, 1978. Investigators ... found that an unlicensed medical technician employed by Small ... had administered a large dose of a dangerous anaesthetic called Innovar to Mrs Plock ... Mrs Plock went into cardiac and respiratory crisis during the operation. Small tried to revive her, and the Board of Medical Quality Assurance [of California] questioned whether his office had the correct emergency equipment.

During the nine-hour period in which Mrs Plock was kept at Small's office after the emergency, a Small employee went to another doctor's office in the same building to ask if he could borrow a tank of oxygen.

Eventually, Small called an ambulance to hospitalise Mrs Plock. Five days later, she died.

The same article reported that Dr Small also attempted a thigh-lift operation, a surgical procedure he had never tried before or even observed. He had read a single article on the subject in a medical journal, but agreed to do the operation anyway. The patient spent five days in Small's office, living on take-out food brought in by his staff, after it became clear the operation (for which he had charged her about £1,400) had failed. When she sought other medical assistance, the diagnosis was that she had gangrene and deep erosion of the tissues in her thighs.

In the June 1979 issue of *Over 21*, writer Mary Davis Peters advises anyone considering surgery at a commercial clinic not to proceed without 'demanding and *getting in writing* the name of the surgeon who would do the work. And I would then ask my doctor to check his qualifications and experience.'

A plastic surgeon suggests, 'Find out where the surgeon was trained, what his qualifications are, what his NHS appointment is, and whether he's a member of the Royal College of Surgeons. If he doesn't have an NHS hospital appointment, there are two possible reasons: either he's a brilliant cosmetic surgeon and doing so well in private that he doesn't need a hospital appointment, *or* he couldn't make the grade in conventional medicine and get a hospital appointment. I'd be very sure which category he was in before I'd let him operate on me.'

In addition to knowledge about the surgeon's training, there are other questions to ask about him or her and about the clinic. How often has the surgeon performed this operation? When was the last time? In surgery, as in most other endeavours, practice makes perfect. In Massachusetts recently, doctors at four hospitals were told they could no longer perform open-heart surgery, because they didn't do the operation often enough to retain their competence and, according to statistics on such surgery, the death rate among their patients was much higher than the norm.

You'll also want information about treatment in case of an emergency. As one plastic surgeon says, 'If everything goes fine, you don't need anything—all you need is a couple of instruments. But you've got to anticipate the unknown.' He recommends that a patient visit the clinic beforehand to find out if they have the following emergency equipment in their operating theatre: a defibrillator (a device to correct abnormal heartbeats); an electrocardiograph; a continuous blood pressure monitor; oxygen; suction equipment to remove excess blood and secretions from the airway; emergency equipment to 'breathe' artificially for a patient; emergency drugs; and emergency lighting in the operating theatre.

Finally, be sure to know what hospital you would be admitted to in case of serious complications.

Surgeons say that the best way to ensure safe and effective plastic surgery is to have a referral from a GP whom you trust. The GP can send you to a surgeon whose work he or she knows, or to the specialist at the closest hospital with a plastic surgery unit.

In theory, no specialist of any kind should see a patient without a referral from a general practitioner. This tradition leads to another problem for some people who want cosmetic surgery—the reluctance of some GPs, particularly older, more traditional ones, to refer patients for such surgery.

Both physicians and plastic surgeons defend the practice of a patient's coming to a specialist through referral by a GP. 'The GP is the guardian of the patient's interest. He knows the plastic surgeon, or he knows him by repute. He is also the guardian of the surgeon's interests. He is unlikely to refer someone who is totally

29

psychologically unsuitable, or for whom such surgery is contraindicated through a medical condition or through drugs they may be taking.'

Sometimes, plastic surgeons say, GPs have refused referrals with such comments as, 'We're in the business of treating sick people, and patients who want such referrals aren't really sick.' Fortunately, this attitude is dying out. There are, however, legitimate grounds on which a GP will refuse to issue a referral. One GP, who is very sympathetic to requests for cosmetic surgery, refused a referral to a woman who was taking steroids for the control of rheumatoid arthritis. 'I tried to make her understand that with any condition requiring long-term steroid treatment, the tissues don't heal that well and so we don't advise cosmetic surgery.'

However, if your health is good and still your GP is reluctant to refer you to a plastic surgeon, then you might want to seek another GP.

Alix Kirsta believes that Britain's medical profession must be educated so that GPs will take requests for cosmetic surgery more seriously than some do. 'Claire Rayner, the agony columnist for the *Sun*, spoke at a meeting of plastic surgeons. She said that a very large proportion of the many letters she gets have to do with plastic surgery. She told about a letter she'd got from a woman who went to a GP about something patently wrong in the structure of a physical feature. He said, "Don't worry. It's not cancer," and sent her home. The surgeons at the meeting said they didn't realise so many women wanted plastic surgery, but they refused to change the GP referral system.'

Rather than change GPs, you can simply go direct to a plastic surgeon. Many surgeons do not turn away patients who come without a referral letter. A London plastic surgeon explains, 'In these cases I write to the GP. I tell him, "This patient came to see me, unsolicited, and I think that I can help her if you have no objections; if you know of any contraindications to surgery, would you be kind enough to let me know. You might prefer to have her referred to another plastic surgeon of your choice who you feel might be able to help her better." I've never had them write back and say no. Most of them don't write back at all.'

How to find the name of a reputable plastic surgeon without going through a GP? Probably the best way is by word of mouth from a friend whose judgement you trust, preferably one who has had an operation done by the surgeon in question. Should you let it be known that you're interested in cosmetic surgery, you may be surprised at the number of people who are also interested or who know someone who has had cosmetic surgery. In fact it's not unusual for people to schedule their surgery for the same time as a friend's so they can keep one another's spirits up in hospital and during convalescence.

If you have friends who work in areas related to show business, modelling, theatre, or beauty, ask them. Cosmetic surgery is an everyday matter among people who rely on their looks to make their living. Perhaps you have a friend who's a nurse or who works in a health-related field. He or she probably has access to names of reliable plastic surgeons.

Especially if you get the name of a plastic surgeon through someone other than a GP, you should check the recommended surgeon in *The Medical Directory*. (Local libraries have copies.) The directory contains information about surgeons' training and appointments. For the best chance of success with the surgery, you'll want a consultant plastic surgeon, preferably at an NHS hospital, who is a member of the Royal College of Surgeons, which means that he or she has the diploma requisite for specialist care. If the surgeon does not have a current appointment at an NHS hospital or is not a member of the RCS, these are good reasons to be cautious and to keep searching for a plastic surgeon.

Another alternative is to send a letter, addressed 'Specialist, Plastic Surgery Unit', to the hospital convenient for you that has such a unit.

As stated earlier, though, generally the best method of finding a cosmetic surgeon is to ask your own GP for a referral. He or she will know things about the surgeons

31

that only another medical professional could find out. If you have been seeing your GP for a while, he or she will be able to take your personality and possible anxieties (about injections, anaesthesia, the surgery itself) into consideration when making a referral.

Many people want to pass up their GP because of embarrassment. In some cases they know their GP socially and would feel uncomfortable revealing their wish for a face lift or a breast augmentation. Even if they don't know their GP on a personal level, they may be embarrassed to be thought so vain and selfish as to ask for unnecessary surgery.

It's probably of little use to say that there is no reason to feel embarrassed. Are you embarrassed to ask a carpenter to remodel your house? Or to have an expensive dress altered so that it fits properly? The desire to have yourself and the things around you look as attractive as possible is normal.

If reluctance to face your GP tempts you to ring up one of the referral services or to visit one of the advertised commercial clinics, balance the five or ten minutes of embarrassment you may feel on confiding in your GP against the risk of having your health endangered, or a permanent or long-term change in your appearance botched, by an incompetent or untrained surgeon.

Chances are very good that if you see your own GP, you will be referred to a qualified, reputable plastic surgeon who will perform cosmetic surgery you'll be satisfied with.

4 The Consultation

A good surgeon must have an eagle's eye, a lion's heart, and a lady's hand.—proverb

A responsible plastic surgeon will insist on a full, lengthy consultation before the surgery. (At some commercial clinics the consultation may be perfunctory, and it may be with someone other than the surgeon who will operate. In some cases you don't even see the surgeon until just before the operation—if then.)

Plastic surgeons emphasise that they are very careful in selecting patients for cosmetic surgery. One estimates that 'ten to fifteen percent of the people seeking cosmetic surgery have serious psychological problems. We try very hard to weed such people out. They won't be pleased no matter how successful the surgery is, and they may sue the surgeon or even take personal revenge by slashing his tyres or dumping paint over his car.'

The surgeon sums up what he's looking for when a patient comes for a consultation: 'As a physician I have to be able to see what the patient is complaining of—in other words, that the problem really does exist. I have to satisfy myself that the patient has thought about the blemish and expects some benefit, but not *too* much—such as a marriage being rebuilt—as the result of a face lift.

'The first questions I ask are always medical, because we have to rule out any physical problem that might make the surgery unwise. If I have medical records from a GP, they often suffice; otherwise I need to take a complete medical history and probably give a physical examination.

33

I'm also interested in chronic medical problems the patient may have, any medication he or she may be taking regularly, and any history of allergies—especially to medication I might plan to use. I'll also want to check blood pressure.

'Some patients are just better candidates for surgery than others because of health, skin condition, bone structure, and outlook.'

Surgeons should ask whether you have had surgery previously, so they can learn whether you tend to bleed excessively, how quickly you heal, and whether you are prone to problems with scars.

The two types of scars that can cause problems are hypertrophic scars and keloids. A hypertrophic scar is a large, raised scar that usually softens and fades with time. Like the hypertrophic scar, a keloid is large and raised, but it spreads beyond the margin of the wound and sometimes continues to grow. People with dark skin are more prone to keloids than fair skinned people; they can be a considerable problem for black people and Orientals seeking surgery. (For more on these scars, see the chapter on scar revision.)

Assuming that you are physically healthy, the surgeon will then be most concerned that your motives are sound and your expectations realistic. He or she may ask what may seem rather personal and irrelevant questions. Adriana Clark was surprised at the length and personal nature of the interview she had with the surgeon. 'He asked me things that would never have occurred to me. What was my husband's attitude? Was anything wrong in our private lives? Was I hoping to become more beautiful to attract him more? Was our marriage in trouble? Things like that. He didn't ask for any details, but for the first time I realised that there are probably people who go for surgery for those reasons. I simply thought nose surgery would be like getting a wonderful new hairdo that I'd have for my whole life.'

Alix Kirsta tells of a friend, an actor, who consulted a plastic surgeon about his nose: he wanted to be able to play a larger variety of roles. 'The surgeon—who is one of

Britain's best—grilled him for two hours to make absolutely sure that his motive was the work as an actor.'

Although, ultimately, the surgeon will determine how much and in what way the surgery will change you, he or she will probably want to know specifically what you think is wrong with the feature you want altered. People with vague, general complaints that they don't like a given feature are often poor risks for cosmetic surgery. They probably are displeased with themselves generally and would not be made happier by one operation—or more, though they may keep shopping for satisfaction through surgery.

There is some controversy about whether it's advisable for surgeons to show prospective patients before-and-after photographs of work they have done on others. Many surgeons don't, because such a review can lead you to unrealistic expectations and to demands for particular alterations that aren't possible or even desirable, given your particular features, skin type, and bone structure.

Some surgeons do, however, have former patients who will answer questions of prospective patients about the surgery they plan. Patients often find that those who have had the operation can understand their concerns in a special way. In particular, women considering breast surgery often feel more comfortable having other women answer their questions.

To be sure the patient makes a well-reasoned judgement about having cosmetic surgery, one plastic surgeon says, 'I won't even let patients make an appointment for surgery during our consultation. I tell them what I can and can't do and find out if the results of the surgery will match what they expect. I tell them about whatever scars there may be. Some people think there won't be any scars, but any time you cut the body, there's scarring. In most operations, we can put the scars in an unobtrusive place, but there will be—and remain—scars from the incision.

'After I've told them what I can do, I tell them to think about it for a week or more and call me if they decide to have the surgery. I want to be sure that they feel under no pressure to make a decision and understand that I'm not

35

"selling" them the operation in any way.

'On that first visit I want to see who they are, what they're like, why they want it done, and whether they need it doing. If they have a stable reason for wanting the surgery, I'll tell them what I can do, where the incisions are made, and something of the serious or potentially serious problems associated with the procedure. I then ask them to go away and think about it, and come back to see me again.'

So much for the surgeon's viewpoint on a consultation. What about you, the patient? The consultation is an opportunity for you to find out whether you trust the surgeon, what happens during the surgery, and what the aftermath will be. You are, after all, purchasing a service; you have every right to know what you are going to get for your money.

Often surgeons don't volunteer enough information, so it's a good idea to bring a list of questions, a notebook, and a pen. Besides writing down the answers to your questions, you might want to take notes on other things the surgeon says to you about the operation. Many surgeons say that patients frequently forget what they were told in the consultation.

Don't be shy about asking questions. Any responsible surgeon will take the time and trouble to answer your questions fully. If not, there is reason to question whether you've come to the right person. One plastic surgeon says, 'The surgeon has to transmit the feeling that the patient is the most important thing facing him at that moment. But if he's on the phone with his accountant or interrupts to make a golf date, that detracts from the rapport there should be in a patient-surgeon relationship and can be an omen that things aren't going to work out.'

Something else a surgeon might do that should make caution signs light up in your head is to suggest additional surgical procedures. If you go to see a surgeon about a nose alteration, don't leave the consulting rooms having agreed to three additional procedures. A surgeon who suggests additional surgery may be more interested in your wallet than in your welfare.

There are two exceptions to this rule. One is the chin implant. Many people who seek nose surgery don't know about the procedure—a very simple one that can aid enormously in balancing the profile when the nose is reshaped. The second exception is eyelid surgery. Some people who see a surgeon about a face lift believe that the lift will take care of bags under the eyes and drooping eyelids. That isn't so, and surgeons will usually mention this if the patient clearly believes that a face lift will take care of all sagging facial skin.

With these suggestions in mind, you're ready to ask the surgeon some questions of your own before you commit yourself to surgery:

- How long will I be in hospital?
- What kind of anaesthesia will be used?
- How much pain will there be, and how is it controlled?
- How long will it take the scars to fade? How detectable or obtrusive will the faded scars be?
- Will there be bruising? Swelling? For how long?
- What are the possible complications of the surgery?
- Will activities be restricted for a period of time after the surgery? How long? (Such information can help you to plan for time off work and for child care.)

If you do not already know about the surgeon's training and hospital appointments, now is a good time to find out. Probably the most important questions to ask at the consultation are:

- How recently and how often has the surgeon done the procedure?
- What complications have the patients experienced?

The last question is one of the most important; a responsible surgeon will discuss in detail the possible complications of the surgery. Any procedure in which an incision is made into the body can lead to any of three possible complications: development of a haematoma, infection, and skin slough. A haematoma, a swelling containing blood, is the most common complication after surgery. If one is going to develop, it usually appears in the first forty-eight hours after surgery. Small haematomas usually disappear within a few weeks. With some larger ones, surgeons can suction off the blood, but in other cases they must operate to remove the blood.

Infections are another possible complication following surgery; the type and severity of the infection will determine the treatment and the length of time it will take to recover from it. Some infections are easily cleared up with penicillin or antibiotics. But more virulent infections can use penicillin as food and even thrive on it. If the infection is resistant to treatment, the period of recuperation may be prolonged (see the case of Caitlin Williams in the breast reduction chapter; she spent almost ten weeks recuperating from an infection after her surgery).

A third possible complication is skin slough following the death of skin around the incision. If the blood supply to the area has been cut off and oxygen cannot get into the tissue, the skin dies of suffocation and turns black. The surgeon will cut out the dead tissue. If the area in which the skin has died is small, the edges of the healthy skin may be brought together; if it is large, surgeons must use skin grafts.

If you are satisfied with the surgeon's answers to your questions and with other information gleaned during the consultation, you have a good chance of being happy with the results of the surgery.

If you decide to go through with the surgery, you'll probably be advised to take some precautions before the operation. Smokers anticipating facial surgery would be well advised to quit, because smoking hinders blood circulation in the skin, an important factor in healing. The surgeon will probably also ask that you not take aspirin for two weeks before the procedure. A single aspirin can prevent normal blood clotting for as long as two weeks.

Finally, the surgeon may suggest that, whatever the specific operation you're having, you not plan any travel by plane during the first two to three weeks after the surgery, because a pressure change inside the plane could rupture an incision. Such a complication is unlikely, but should it occur, you're out of reach of immediate medical attention.

The journey that begins with the thought, 'I'd like to have my nose done' and ends in an operating theatre isn't an easy one. But the more care you take with each step, the better your chance to have safe and effective cosmetic surgery.

5 A Note on Anaesthesia

... a soft numbness diffuses all my inmost senses with deep oblivion.—Horace

Before scheduling your cosmetic surgery, you and your surgeon must determine what form of anaesthesia to use: local or general. For most operations, there is a choice; others (such as breast reduction and abdomen surgery) must be done under general anaesthetic.

Most plastic surgery in Britain is done under general anaesthetic. Even American doctors, who are very proud of their standards, admit that Britain has a greater percentage of skilled anaesthetists and thus a far higher standard of general anaesthesia.

Some patients, surgeons say, insist upon general anaesthetic, because they don't want to know what is happening to them during the surgery. Others frightened of losing consciousness, request local anaesthetic. A few say they are indifferent to the type of anaesthetic used and would leave the choice to the surgeon. Where there is a choice of anaesthesia and the patient has a preference, the surgeon should take those wishes into consideration.

The reason that British general anaesthesia is considered so good is that it lowers the blood pressure, giving the surgeon better operating conditions. Either of two drugs can be injected intravenously to lower blood pressure; another is used as an inhaled anaesthetic agent.

In Britain only a qualified physician can administer general anaesthesia; there are not nurse/anaesthetists as there are in some other countries.

Many anaesthetists and plastic surgeons assert that plastic surgeons are very careful in their choices of anaesthetists and work only with those who are both well qualified and experienced.

A plastic surgeon says, 'I much prefer operating on a patient who has had general anaesthetic. I work with an anaesthetist I trust, which means that I can concentrate totally on the operation and ignore everything else. With a local, I have to keep asking the patient, "Is that all right?" or "Does it hurt?" Like most surgeons, I prefer to administer local anaesthetic myself, and in a long operation I have to keep reaching for the syringe for the local to reinforce the anaesthetic.'

In deciding what general anaesthetic to use and how to administer it, the anaesthetist will consider the patient's overall general health and past medical history as well as the nature of the operation and the amount of time it will take.

The anaesthetist should see the patient the day before the surgery and explain the procedure. One says, 'I can usually tell in a few minutes' conversation how the patient reacts to stress. I can prescribe a tranquilliser and a preoperative medication if that seems necessary.

'My usual procedure in the operating theatre is to give the patient a quick-acting barbiturate, which puts them to sleep in ten to fifteen seconds. Then I either put a mask over their nose and mouth or a tube down to their lungs and administer the general anaesthetic.'

The most commonly used local anaesthetic is Lidocaine. Preoperative sedation is almost always used before local anaesthetic. Many patients report that with local anaesthetic and sedation they were in a state of euphoria and afterwards remembered nothing that had happened during the operation, though they had responded to the surgeon's requests to sit up, turn, or otherwise move upon request. During a long operation the surgeon will have to inject more of the local anaesthetic to keep you pain free. The advantages of local anaesthetic are that you can usually leave the hospital sooner—perhaps the same day you have surgery—and won't have to pay an anaesthetist's fee.

41

The commercial clinics use local anaesthetic whenever possible. One anaesthetist says, 'In my opinion, they do that to promote turnover. You don't need the same facilities if you're using local anaesthetic.'

Both general and local anaesthetic involve the risk of complications. There is the risk of an overdose with a local anaesthetic, which should be injected only into the tissues. If it is accidentally injected into a vein or artery, it can be taken into the system too quickly. The patient may sweat and feel generally ill or may experience a sudden drop in blood pressure, or may suffer cardiac arrest or an epileptic seizure (even if the patient is not an epileptic).

After a general anaesthetic, some patients experience discomfort because of damage to local tissue if a tube was put through the nose and into the lungs. One result can be a sore throat that lasts for two or three days. It is also possible to have a tooth chipped. And, *extremely* rare though it is, there have been cases of death caused by the faulty administration of general anaesthetic.

The New York *Times* has reported that two of the chemicals which have been used in general anaesthetics, chloroform and trichloroethylene, can damage nerve fibres themselves or the myeline sheath that encases them.

An anaesthetist says, 'There's no problem so long as one knows the dangers and is alert to them. I have never seen a problem with trichloroethylene when it was properly used.' The same anaesthetist admits that if improperly used, real damage can occur. He recounted that certain industrial workers had inhaled a compound in which trichloroethylene was a major ingredient, and it rotted their cranial nerves.

Neither local nor general anaesthesia may be used without risk, and the patient can only make a choice after weighing the advantages and risks of each.

6 It's All Over And . . .

Weeping may endure for a night
but joy cometh in the morning.
—Psalms

It's been ten days since you had a face lift, the surgeon has pronounced the result beautiful—and you feel like crying most of the time. A strange response? Not at all. A feeling of depression is a common reaction, even though cosmetic surgery is often called 'happy surgery'. So don't feel shamefully irrational if you are depressed and weepy for a while afterwards. Allow yourself time to adjust to the new you.

One difficult adaptation was described by a London oral surgeon who operates on jaws. He had corrected the markedly protruding jawline of a young woman, 'and the alteration in her appearance was so great that she was in tears for two or three weeks. She couldn't recognise herself when she looked in the mirror. And it upset her very much, even though, objectively, she looked so much better. After four weeks she said, "I can't stand it anymore. You must put my jaw back where it was." Once the operation's done, it's very difficult to put it back. But I thought that if I took the splints off too soon, a certain amount of relapse would take place; the muscles would pull the jaw back almost to where it had been. She pleaded with me to do it, so I removed the splints. And two weeks later, she was pleading with me *not* to let her jaw go back. By this time, she had mentally readjusted and was delighted with the results. It took her a transition period of about six weeks to get used to her new face. Fortunately,

43

the jaw stayed where I had set it in surgery. Nine times out of ten it would have receded at least somewhat.'

After nose surgery, many patients experience initial disappointment on removal of the plaster seven to ten days after the surgery. Adriana Clark says, 'You think you're going to look immediately different and glamorous, and it will be everything you ever wanted. That wasn't so. I had work done on the bridge of my nose, so the area between my eyes was very swollen, and my nose was just splayed across my face.'

Surgeons say that depression after surgery is often related to the age of the patient. Most people seventeen to twenty—a common age for nose surgery—have little difficulty adjusting, because they don't yet have a fixed image of their body. But it is not uncommon for face lift patients to be depressed for two or three weeks after the surgery. The operation is commonly done on middle-aged people, who have a difficult time revising their mental image of a face they have lived with for so long.

Of course, the biggest problem comes if you remain unhappy with the results of your surgery. That's what happened to actress Daria Young. She went to a man who is now an eminent plastic surgeon in London and who had studied with one of the founders of modern plastic surgery. She recalls, 'He was less skilled than he cared to admit. I was left with a tiny, super-short, slightly ridiculous-looking nose. The nearer I got to forty, the more infantile it seemed. *I* looked more womanly, and *it* looked more childlike.' (While working in the United States for a year, she had her nose operated on again by a surgeon who is considered one of the world's leaders in repairing botched plastic surgery. The results were excellent.)

Surgeons say—and patients bear out—that it's unusual for a patient to be dissatisfied with results that the surgeon finds satisfactory. If both agree that the result is disappointing, a second operation can be arranged after the healing from the first operation is complete. Surgeons normally do not charge for the second operation.

During your period of recuperation, surgeons suggest

that you strike a mean between resuming physical activity too quickly and unnecessarily prolonging the period of convalescence. Relaxation for a week to ten days is helpful after even minor surgery; for major surgery, the period may be even longer. (Exceptions to this are dentistry, electrolysis, and hair transplants, none of which requires a period of convalescence.)

After the first ten days to two weeks of recuperation, many surgeons suggest that you let comfort be your guide to activity. If you feel a sensation of pulling or stretching on your incision, be gentle.

A plastic surgeon says, 'I tell my patients to give themselves a chance to heal, but, barring complications, they should be back to their ordinary routine—including vigorous physical exercise—after a month. I also want them to be on a sound, balanced diet during their convalescence. Good nutrition can promote the healing process.'

Following successful surgery, not long after everything is healed and post-operative swelling or bruising has disappeared, you'll probably forget what you used to look like. Some people say that they have little opportunity to compare their 'old' to their 'new' selves, because they were so self-conscious before the surgery that they had avoided scrutinising themselves in mirrors and wouldn't let anyone photograph them.

Another surprise could come when you resume working and pursuing your ordinary social life. Unless the change in your appearance is thoroughly dramatic, most people who see you regularly won't notice that you've had a specific feature altered. The usual response is, 'Your holiday must have done you good. You look rested.'

Acquaintances who see you infrequently are more likely to notice the specific change than friends, relatives, and work colleagues who see you all the time. People we see regularly tend to see the total person, whereas casual acquaintances may be more conscious of the change in a specific feature.

For the best chance that people won't spot your

45

cosmetic surgery, here's a tip from several patients who have had different kinds of facial surgery done: just before you return to work, have your hair cut or styled in a different way. Most people will attribute your overall change to the new hairstyle. Of course, there are some operations, such as hair transplants or a very pronounced change in profile, that can't be disguised.

Most patients say that returning to work and social life after cosmetic surgery was far easier than they had expected, because they had been more conscious than others of the body part they'd had corrected.

7 Paying for Cosmetic Surgery

Let the world slide, let the world go:
A fig for care, and a fig for woe!
If I can't pay, why I can owe ...
  —John Heywood

Because most cosmetic surgery is elective—not undertaken for physical health reasons—it is usually done privately rather than on the NHS. But if you can convince your GP that some feature is bothering you enough to prompt a psychological problem, he or she may decide that the operation would contribute significantly to your mental health and so recommend that it be done on the NHS. The plastic surgeon, however, need not accept the GP's recommendation. Says one, 'Some aesthetic [cosmetic] work is done under NHS. At present, the vast majority of NHS hospitals have far too few facilities to take in aesthetic work, or the waiting list is years long.'

Plastic surgeons may not feel that they can justify using scarce NHS resources for such surgery—or they may just be greedy. Polly Toynbee quoted a plastic surgeon in the *Guardian*:

To be truly honest, which most doctors aren't, why should I take a client on the NHS when I can make a lot of money making him come to me privately? It would be entirely my decision as to whether to treat someone for a new nose in my NHS hospital, but I always turn them down and say they must see me privately. Anyone can afford it if they save, as they might for a new car.

47

That cavalier attitude is balanced by the sympathy of many other plastic surgeons, who will perform the surgery under NHS if they believe that the patient genuinely can't afford it and that the surgery could make a real difference in the patient's feeling of psychological well-being. One comments, 'I think people should pay who can afford it. But if they can't, and if I believe it's really important to them, I'll do it on the NHS. Besides, I like doing the surgery.'

The cost of private plastic surgery (see Appendix: Costs) includes more than the surgeon's fee. There is also a fee for the anaesthetist if you are having general anaesthesia (usually ten to twenty-five per cent of the surgeon's fee), the charge for the operating theatre, the hospital or nursing home cost, and the fees for drugs and dressings.

Some plastic surgeons require full payment in advance for work done privately. They offer a variety of arguments for this practice, but the substance is that the surgeons fear patients may change their minds before the surgery. The surgeons have blocked out the time in their schedules and have engaged an operating theatre and an anaesthetist; they have to pay those costs even if patients change their minds. Unlike other surgery, whose cancellation jeopardises a patient's health, there is nothing life-threatening in a decision not to go through with planned cosmetic surgery.

If you can afford to pay and have the cash on hand, you're all set. If you don't have the cash, what are the options? You can maintain a rigorous savings programme for two or three years. (Beverly Hall, who wanted her nose altered, took a second job on weekend evenings at the local cinema, put that money into a special savings account, and was able to have her surgery after eighteen months.) However, with inflation creeping or vaulting ever upwards, you may find that an operation that cost £700 when you began saving costs £800 by the time you have accrued the £700.

Many people would prefer to have the surgery now and pay for it over two or three years, while enjoying the results. One of the attractions of some commercial clinics is that they offer such financing. However, if you would prefer not to undertake the other risks that surgery at a clinic often brings, and if you have good credit and a valuable asset for collateral (house, property, car), you might consider a bank loan.

Bank managers say they wouldn't care what your purpose is in wanting the loan; their concern is only whether you are a good risk for paying the money back. Most say that they would not lend the entire sum, that the client should show good faith by putting up a portion of the amount needed. They will check your credit, but no one else need know the specific reason you want the loan. Bank managers warn that if the money supply is tight, they often have to cut back on all personal loans.

Now that we have covered the general issues involved in cosmetic surgery, let's look at specific operations and what is involved in them.

Procedures

8 Nose Alteration

My beauty is my curse.—Miss Piggy*

TV comedienne-singer Marti Caine knew when she was sixteen that she didn't like her nose, but she was in her thirties before she was able to have it altered. Fortunately, the result has been worth the wait. Here's her story.

'My nose was very long, and it had been broken twice when I was a child. It wasn't so bad while I had a round face. I used to be quite heavy, and my nose looked fine then. But as I lost weight, my nose seemed to become bigger and bigger. In fact, it was my face that was getting smaller and smaller.

'I decided that I could do with a new nose, but I had children growing up, and the money was going elsewhere. I considered taking out an insurance policy that would mature in five years, or maybe getting a bank loan, because I was determined to have it done. As it happened, I "made it" and was able to have the operation without money being a problem.

'I finally made the decision after seeing myself on television for the first time. I was a nose on legs. It was long and thin, and the end of it cast a shadow over my top lip. I looked like Hitler. I couldn't believe it. When you look at yourself in the mirror, you tend not to see a bad point. Photographs tell the truth, but I kidded myself that they were bad photographs. I had spent hours and hours

*Star of Jim Henson's Muppets.

53

experimenting with make up to disguise my nose. But lighting on television shows it up, and there's no way to hide it.

'I would have had my nose altered even if I had not been a performer. It had nothing to do with my profession. I'd like to be able to say that I did it for professional reasons, but that would be an out-and-out lie. I did it from vanity—sheer feminine vanity.

'When I went for the consultation with the surgeon, he said he could correct the length. I had expected him to show me pictures of various noses and ask which one I'd like, but he didn't. I didn't have any choice. He said, "Don't expect miracles, because there's a bend in your nose, and it's going to stay there because it suits your face." He said he wanted my nose to look like a real nose, not like a doll's.

'To shorten the tip of my nose, he had to take away my flared nostrils. I liked them, because I could demonstrate my anger with them beautifully, and I miss them dreadfully.

'I went into hospital the evening before the operation and left the day after. I went in before to make sure I didn't have anything to eat. They asked me if I wanted a sedative the night before, but I refused. I wasn't in the least bit nervous; I probably could have slept on a clothesline.

'The next morning at eleven, they put me to sleep in my bed. I had a general anaesthetic—as long as I don't know about it, I don't care what they do. I would have had a local if I'd had to; I wanted my nose done so badly I would have let them do it without anything. I woke up a couple of hours later, and I felt normal—just like I do now—except that my mouth was coated with blood and was very, very dry.

'The only discomfort I had came with the first drink of water. Because my nose was plugged up, I had a sort of drowning sensation with the first swallow. But I was amazed at how painless the whole thing was.

'The next day I left hospital and went home. During the week I had the plaster on, I stayed inside. I didn't want anyone to see me, or to know, until it was ready and I could say, "Well, what do you think?"

'After the first day, I did have bruising. I started to go black from the corners of my nose downwards, even under my chin. It went from a nice blue to a deep purple and from deep purple to glorious yellow. Seven days later when I went to London to have the pot [the plaster cast] removed, the swelling on my face was subsiding, but there was still some bruising.

'The biggest disappointment came when the surgeon took the pot off the week after the operation. I was dying to know what it looked like. He took the bandage off and said, "Beautiful." And I looked at myself in the mirror and was horrified. I've not cried since I was seven, but I felt like crying. There was no indentation. My nose was just straight across. Now I looked like Kermit the Frog. And the surgeon was beside himself with glee because it was so wonderful. I thought, Is he having me on, or what?

'When I went home after having the pot off, my kids were waiting to see what I looked like. Their chins began to quiver when they saw me. My youngest son came up with the consolation, "Well, never mind, mother; you're a comic."

'Our next-door neighbours hadn't seen me for a week. The husband was out cutting the lawn when I came home. He caught a glimpse of me through the window, and all he could see were black eyes and a swollen face. He wouldn't speak to my husband; he thought he'd hit me.

'After two weeks I realised that I really liked it, although first thing in the morning, it was a little more swollen than it was at the end of the day. It took a good year for it to settle down to what it is now—which is normal. By the time the swelling had gone down, the kids had forgotten what I looked like before, and so had my husband. As far as I'm concerned, I've always looked like this.

'When I first went to see my two very best friends, nothing was said for the first half hour. Finally I asked, "Well? Do you notice anything different?" They said, 'You've put weight on? You've had your hair cut? You've plucked your eyebrows?" They went through a whole list of things, and finally I had to tell them I had had my nose altered. Your close friends won't see it, but people who don't know you very well will see it straightaway, because they see the physical you, whereas your friends and relatives see the personality.

'After I had my nose done, I could wear my hair any way I wanted. I could wear it up, and I could sit in profile, which I had hated doing. I would catch sight of myself in shop doorways and say, "That's me"... I was so amazed at the difference.

'I think people in the public eye won't talk about their cosmetic surgery because they want people to think they've been like that all the time, or they're afraid of being thought vain. Well, I *am* vain. Everybody's vain. Otherwise I wouldn't bother with deodorants, or shaving my legs, or plucking my eyebrows. The operation helped me as a person to look better, and I'm hoping to help others in a roundabout way.

'I wish to God I'd had it done years ago, had the surgeons been as expert as they are now. It made such a difference to me as a woman; I became a more sexual, less aggressive person. If I'd had my nose done ten years ago, I wouldn't have the personality that I have now.

'I have the personality of a plain person, which I used to attract males: "She's a good laugh, a good giggle, one of the lads." That was a deliberate image choice when I was younger, and it got me all the guys I wanted. I listened to all the best radio programmes with comedy on them and found the best time to use the funny lines. I was a must for every party, and I became a leader. I wouldn't have otherwise, because I was skinny, and I didn't have the clothes.

'I still have that personality, because I lived so long with the old nose. But my new personality is just beginning to come out: one of being less a tomboy—less one of the lads— and being more a female, feminine-type woman.'

Dorothy Smedley lives alone in a small town in Kent. She is now forty-eight and works as a nurse. Like Marti Caine, she had been self-conscious about her nose for many years before she was able to have an operation. However, the

results for her weren't so happy as they were for Marti
Caine, and her experience shows the necessity of dealing
with a reputable surgeon.

'I'd been very self-conscious about my nose, because it
had become rather bulbous at the tip. Although I'd been
very humorous about it, I'd often thought about plastic
surgery. But this was not for me; it was for people with
money. Just about the time I had some superannuation
coming, I saw an advert in a paper for a cosmetic clinic.
Things had gone a bit wrong for me and I was a bit low, so
I decided to spend the money I'd got on having my nose
done. I telephoned the advert number and spoke to Mr M.
He said he would send me the brochure, which he did.
Then an appointment was made for me at his clinic in
north London.

'When I went there, Mr M introduced me to Mr B. I
learned later that he was a doctor with a background in
general surgery. He examined my nose and said that he
could shorten the tip and refine the bulbousness of it,
which is what I wanted. We arranged a date, and I paid Mr
M for the operation. Then he had a professional
photographer come in and take pictures of me.

'When I got to the clinic for the operation, I suppose I
noticed more than most, because I'm a nurse. My first
impression was that people were being wheeled in and out
of the operating theatre very fast. And I did find it strange
that they didn't ask me if I had washed my face before they
took me.

'They used a local anaesthetic, so I was aware of what
was going on. I couldn't feel any pain, although there was
this terrible crunch on the bridge of my nose.

'A week after the operation I went back to have the
plaster removed from my nose. Obviously, it was very
swollen and very bruised. Mr B said it would take about
fifteen days for the bruising to go away. Three weeks later
I noticed this lump on the bridge of my nose, which I had
never had before. The bridge had been perfectly straight.

'I tried to reach Mr M, but it took several phone calls and
a letter before he spoke to me. In the letter I said that I was
a nurse, that I worked terribly hard for my money, and that

57

I was very disappointed. He made an appointment for me to see Mr B. I said that the tip was still the same; the bulbousness was still there. Mr B said he couldn't do anything for six months. Then he operated to refine the tip, but he wouldn't touch the bridge of my nose, even though it had been perfectly straight before.

'When I went home, I had just a little plaster on the tip. A week after it was taken off, an infection broke out. I woke up and this terrible pus was coming from my nose, and the nose had completely collapsed—there's no cartilage left in it. The pus lasted for nearly a year.

'I went to see Mr B. He gave me a tetracycline ointment, but it didn't work. Then I went to my GP. I was very embarrassed, because they are dealing with illnesses and problems that are real. He took a swab and found I had a staphylococcus infection—an infection often picked up by patients while they're in a hospital. I finally went to a dermatologist, but it took eleven months to clear up the infection.

'In the meantime I saw a television programme with Mr M talking about how they could get rid of all sorts of facial lines. It made me so angry. After that I went to my solicitors. I didn't want to be vindictive, and I didn't want money or anything. All I wanted was my nose put back right. I was so self-conscious and depressed about it.

'Mr M didn't even answer my solicitor's letter until the medical officer from Camden visited him.

'Now I'm seeing a plastic surgeon I found through my dermatologist; he will give me an expert opinion on the condition of my nose for the solicitors. Then they'll tell me exactly what they can do to put this right.'*

The most commonly requested cosmetic surgery in the world is alteration of the nose—rhinoplasty—and it almost seems there are as many reasons for the request as

---

*It is the impression of the plastic surgeon consulted by Ms Smedley that the English plastic surgery community regards Mr M as 'a fraud' and Mr B as a 'butcher'. However, he also believes that for Dorothy Smedley to pursue legal remedies could be ruinously expensive and that the chances of collecting from Mr M and Mr B would be almost nil because of the maze of legal technicalities sure to be raised.

there are people who make it. British actress Daria Young was told that her career wouldn't take off until she was forty and had 'grown into' her nose. Then she'd be ready for character parts. 'I thought,' she says, 'that I had a modest talent and a light voice, so that I had to have my career while I was young. I decided when I came to London to study acting that I would have my nose bobbed.'

Cosmetician Janet Lowell was embarrassed by the large tip of her nose and felt especially humiliated when after-dinner drinks were served at a party. 'My nose was so bulbous that I always ended up with some of the liqueur on the tip of it.'

And secretary Adriana Clark got fed up with comparisons to Barbra Streisand. 'When people wanted to be kind, they'd say, "You look just like Barbra Streisand." Or sometimes they'd say I looked like Liza Minnelli. I had a very strong, very aggressive nose, and since I'm an aggressive person, I didn't need the nose to announce it.'

Fortunately for these women, and for other people who would like a nose with a different shape, the nose is easier to modify than many other body parts, because so much of it is made of cartilage—firm but flexible tissue.

While nose surgery is frequently done simply for cosmetic reasons, it may also be done to correct breathing difficulties caused by a deviated septum. If health considerations are involved, the surgery can be done on NHS.

Because noses are so individual and varied, there are a number of corrections possible:

- A large nose can be reduced by removing cartilage.
- A long nose can be shortened by removing cartilage and soft tissue.
- Too-small noses can be increased in size with implants.
- The line of the nose can be narrowed.
- A bump can be removed.
- The tip can be shortened or reduced in size.
- The droop of the tip associated with middle age can be corrected.

The surgeon aims to give you a nose that conforms with the rest of your face, while providing a well-defined tip, an angle between the nose and the lip of ninety to ninety-five degrees, and a pleasing triangular shape to the base (where the nostrils are).

Consultation

The surgeon will examine your nose and tell you what he or she can and can't do. Some surgeons take a Polaroid photo and trace the planned revision on it. For the more important medical photographs to be used in planning and, as is often the case, during the actual surgery, you may be sent to a professional medical photographer; or the surgeon may take such photos. You'll be lying down during the operation, so the photos are needed for reference to what your nose looks like when you're standing or seated.

No reputable surgeon will promise a nose like one you've seen in a photograph or admired on your favourite rock star or film idol; in fact a sure way to make a surgeon wary of operating on your nose is to arrive with a picture of the nose you want. That nose may be all wrong for your face, or even impossible to achieve, given your bone structure and certain properties of your skin. If you have been careful in your search for a reputable specialist and trust your surgeon to do a competent job, you very probably should also trust her or his judgement in fitting your new nose to your face.

At the consultation the surgeon may suggest a chin implant to balance your new profile. This is a simple procedure that adds little in time or cost to the surgery.

Preferred Age

Nasal surgery is usually associated with people in their late teens and twenties, though it can be done on older people. The operation is performed only after the nasal bone has completed its growth. For girls, that's usually fifteen to sixteen; and for boys, who mature more slowly, the minimum age is usually seventeen or eighteen. The optimum age is between sixteen and thirty, because the skin during those years will be best for draping over the reshaped nose.

Hospitalisation

How long you're in a hospital or clinic will depend on several factors, principally whether you have local or general anaesthesia. Adriana Clark had local anaesthetic and came home a couple of hours after the operation. Though she herself had little discomfort, she wishes that she had stayed overnight to avoid the scare she gave her family when she began bleeding soon after she arrived home.

If you and the surgeon choose general anaesthesia, it's likely, barring complication, that you will be able to leave the hospital one or two days after the operation.

Anaesthesia

The operation can be done under local anaesthetic, with preoperative sedation, but many surgeons—and patients —prefer general anaesthetic.

Procedure

You will be instructed to scrub your face with antiseptic solution the night before the surgery, and your face will be scrubbed again in the operating theatre. The hairs in your nose will be clipped so that dried blood doesn't collect on them.

All incisions are made inside the nose. After separating the skin from the bone and cartilage that form the skeleton of the nose, the surgeon proceeds to make the necessary correction according to the plan designed before the surgery.

To remove a bump or correct a hooked, crooked, or

wide nose, surgeons use small surgical saws or chisels under the skin of the nose. They fracture the nasal bones and reset them. To correct a saddle nose, which has a large depression in the bridge, the surgeon fills in the depression with cartilage, bone, or a silicone implant.

A nose that is too short can be lengthened by adding bone or implanting silicone under the skin covering the existing nose bone.

To change a bulbous tip, the surgeon will refashion the four pieces of cartilage that support and shape the tip.

The surgeon will not know the final result until the skin is draped over the refashioned nose. Heavy, turgid skin doesn't drape well and the tissues won't accommodate the new shape.

If you are black, your surgery will probably involve raising the nose bridge, using either cartilage from your body or plastic material. For a result that will please the black patient and suit other facial features, it's often necessary to decrease the size of the nostrils. This is done by removing tissue at the outer corner of each nostril. Surgeons find that black skin is especially difficult to work on at the nose where it tends to be very thick.

The operation takes about one hour.

Aftermath

When you wake up after the operation, you'll have plugs in your nose. They are usually removed within twenty-four to forty-eight hours after the operation. During that time you'll have to breathe through your mouth, which can make it difficult to swallow solid food; some people find it easiest to eat very soft foods, such as baby food. Adriana Clark had a very dry throat the morning after the operation because she had been breathing through her mouth all night. Like many people, Adriana felt greatly relieved when the packing came out; but after fifteen or twenty minutes she experienced swelling in the soft tissues. Her surgeon prescribed nose drops, which she used at regular intervals to ease the obstruction.

There will be a plaster cast on your nose to protect it,

and a bandage across that. These will come off in a week to ten days.

There will probably be bruising around your nose and just below your eyes; that can take from a week to ten days to clear up.

Adriana Clark's eyeballs turned red for a few days after the operation. Her surgeon explained that this reaction is not uncommon and is caused by blood escaping from the nasal area during and after surgery. The condition disappeared without treatment, as he said it would.

Swelling of the face, discolouration, and swelling of the eyelids should disappear within seven to fourteen days. The swelling of the nose itself will disappear sometime between three months and a year after the operation. A plastic surgeon says, 'We don't know very much about swelling and the reasons that it settles down more quickly in some persons than in others. As a rule of thumb, we say that after a rhinoplasty you have eighty-five per cent of your final result in a month, ninety-five per cent in six months, and one hundred per cent in a year.'

Daria Young experienced numbness inside her nose for several months after her operation; this also is to be expected.

If the surgery is done properly, there should be no pain. Afterwards you should feel as though you have a heavy cold. Some patients report that having the bandage removed a week or so after the operation was painful, but the duration of the pain was mercifully brief.

Convalescence

Most people have little problem returning to work two to three weeks after the operation. Women can mask the remaining effects of the operation with make up.

Your surgeon will want you to rest and to avoid any bending or strain, including that involved even in light housekeeping, for at least the first ten days, because it is important that there be no elevation in the blood pressure. For the first two or three weeks, you'll sleep on your back with your head raised at a forty-five degree angle.

63

After a week or ten days, you should find yourself breathing normally.

You will be asked to restrict strenuous activities for four to six weeks. Usually surgeons prefer that you avoid body-contact sports for about three months so that you won't risk dislocating the nasal bone, which is still healing.

You should avoid blowing your nose at all for the first ten days and be very gentle with it for several weeks after that.

Unfortunately, you'll even have to restrict kissing for the first two to three weeks.

It's very important not to over-expose your 'new' nose to the sun for the first three to six months. The sun assaults tissues and can cause an inflammation reaction in injured tissues; strong sunlight will burn the skin on the nose when the blood supply isn't yet back to normal. If you're going to be in the sun, wear a hat with a visor and apply a sunscreen agent.

People who wear spectacles may have some problems, because for a while you won't be able to wear glasses with heavy frames or with a tight fit at the bridge of the nose. Some surgeons suggest taping eye-glasses to the forehead until you are able to wear them normally (after about ten days). Contact lenses can be worn as soon as eyelid swelling has subsided.

Scars

Incisions are made inside the nose for cosmetic nasal operations, so there are no external scars.

Complications

Cosmetic nose surgery carries few complications. Most common is bleeding from the nose. Such bleeding usually occurs within the first ten days and can be a very frightening experience. Adriana Clark's husband thought that she was having a serious haemorrhage when she began bleeding after he brought her home. One surgeon says that postoperative patients 'can drop a pint of blood on the floor.' The bleeding can usually be stopped easily (often by replacing the packing in the nose), but you should have someone call your surgeon at the first sign.

Occasionally there is infection, which can be treated with antibiotics.

Durability of Result

The result of a nose alteration is permanent. People contemplating rhinoplasty can take comfort in the fact that it's probably the oldest, best-practised branch of cosmetic surgery. Two thousand years before Christ, Hindu potters were constructing noses cut off as punishment of criminal offenders. (The technique they employed, still in modified use, is called 'the Indian flap'.) In the twentieth century, nose surgery is more often performed to correct one of nature's errors or to repair a nose injured in a rugby match. Whatever the reason for the surgery, alteration of the nose can make a major change in the harmony of facial features.

9 Face Lift

Look in my face. My name is Used-to-was;
I am also called Played-out and Done-to-Death.
                                        —Henry Duff Traill

Christine MacKay is an American actress who has lived
and worked in London for twenty years. Until she was
thirty-five, she played young women in their late twenties,
enjoying some success on the London stage; on TV and in
commercials she played women in their thirties. Then the
parts dried up, and Christine realised that she was at an
awkward, in-between age—too old for ingenues and too
young for 'character' parts. She realised that her ageing
face was limiting the kinds of parts being offered to her.

'For professional reasons, I decided I wanted some extra
time before I began playing Shelley Winters parts. When I
first asked about having a face lift, the surgeon—whom I
had known for years—wouldn't do it, because I was ten
pounds overweight.

'When I lost the weight and had the surgery, I spent four
days in a nursing home after the operation, which took
about three hours. I had a local anaesthetic—I was always
awake, but I wasn't in pain. On the second day after the
surgery, I was able to get up, and on the third day some of
the stitches came out. For the first twenty-four hours, I had
to use ice packs all over my face.

'Altogether, I found the experience unpleasant, even
though I'm happy with the results. I wasn't prepared for
the after-effects, which no one tells you about. No one tells
you that you look like a gila monster right after the
operation. Your eyes are swollen shut. You become very

66

numb and can't feel anything—like your ears. It took six months for that numbness to go away; for some people, it takes a year. About two months after I had the surgery, I was drying my hair with a hand-held dryer, and I badly burned the back of my ear because I had no feeling there.

'From the head stitches, I feel the need to wash my hair every day. But, oddly, I don't feel the need to moisturise my skin as I used to, even though it was very dry.

'The results of the surgery were excellent. I feel I have several years ahead of playing younger women. But I can't say the operation was an experience I look forward to going through again.'

The face lift of sixty-year-old Theresa Foot, a buyer for a retail clothing chain, was a mother-daughter affair. Theresa was so apprehensive about the operation that daughter Constance, a forty-year-old writer, was involved in every step, from consultation through convalescence. Both women live in London and are accustomed to moving in circles where looks are an important value. Constance tells her mother's story.

'When I told my mother that I wanted to have my eyes done, but I couldn't afford it, she admitted that she saw herself as a candidate for a face lift. There was puffiness on her upper eyelids and bags under her eyes; they run in our family. Her neck was saggy, and her cheeks were drooping at the bottom.

'She kept talking about it, but she was so scared that she couldn't bring herself to do anything. As she's got older, she's become more dependent upon me. She's had four marriages and now she's alone, supporting my grand-mother. But this wasn't a case of "My husband walked out on me so I'm having my face fixed." I encouraged her to have the lift because I thought it would be good for her morale, and she really needed it physically.

'I heard about a plastic surgeon who was supposed to be very good. I went to see him with the idea that I might have my own eyes done at some point, but really as a scout for my mother.

'I finally got my mother to see the surgeon. He looked at

her and suggested a complete face lift as well as surgery on the upper and lower eyelids. He said that the operation would be done in his clinic; that if she went into hospital the cost would be double.

'To myself I questioned the idea of having major surgery done on this outpatient basis. But I thought, "He knows what he's doing."

'On the morning of the surgery I drove her to the clinic at seven-thirty; I picked her up at three-thirty. She was barely conscious, and her head, including her eyes, was completely bandaged, with slits for her mouth and nose. As I was putting mum into the car, the nurse gave me tons of prescriptions and told me to bring her back in three days.

'I took her home and put her to bed with ice packs, which I kept on constantly. She was dying of thirst, but I'd been told that she was supposed to have just ice in her mouth, and not too much water.

'She had more pain afterwards than we expected, and I found that some of the prescriptions were for painkillers. Early in the evening I noticed blood on the back of the bandage. I thought it was strange, and then I noticed that there was also blood on the pillow. About ten o' clock I went in and checked, and the pillow was soaked in blood. She asked me why I kept waking her up.

'I was so upset that I called the doctor, but he didn't seem concerned at all. I tried to explain to him that the pillow and the pillowcase were soaked in blood. Finally, I said, "I think she's bleeding to death." He said I could bring her to see him in the morning.

'I called my friend Eileen, who came over early in the morning. Mum knew she didn't have to see the doctor for three days, and we wildly made up a story that we'd learned the nurse's instructions had been wrong.

'As we put her in Eileen's car, poor mother had no idea that she was in a bloody nightgown with bloody bandages over her head. Even in this terrible situation I got a laugh: Eileen had a brand-new Mercedes, and she kept telling my mother not to lean back against the seat. Poor mother couldn't understand why, but she obeyed.

68

'When we got her to the surgery, everyone was very blasé, but the surgeon did admit, "Yes, she could have died."

'Mother looked just terrible—swollen and bruised—when the bandages came off after three days. Unfortunately, the nurse who took out the stitches left three stitches in; they festered and became raised scars.

'Mum spent five more days in bed, but after two weeks she was back at work, wearing tinted glasses.

'Fortunately, the story has a happy ending. Mother healed beautifully and now looks terrific—at least ten years younger. She is thrilled with her appearance, despite the fact that she almost died.

'When I've saved enough money for my own cosmetic surgery, I definitely will not go back to that surgeon. His callousness and lack of concern really got to me.'

Fifty-three-year-old Rebecca Wilson lives with her husband and two sons in Cambridge, where her husband is associated with the university library. Rebecca began to study for an advanced degree after some twenty years away from academic work.

'I thought about a face lift for about two years before I had it. The droopier I got, the more I thought. You really notice the signs of ageing over a short period - a year or two. I can certainly tell just looking at myself and friends of mine.

'I never had a good chin line. Then my neck started getting crêpey and awful. People had always said that I looked younger than my age. Suddenly I *did* look my age. And I had just finished a doctorate and was about to start looking for a job. I didn't expect to feel like a new woman after an operation, but I did think I'd look better.

'I started dropping little joking hints to my husband, and I talked it over seriously with a close woman friend. Then I talked to my husband about it. He was very supportive and said that if I wanted to have it done, I should.

'We have a GP I trust completely, and he recommended a surgeon I've been very happy with.

'At the consultation, he gave me a mirror and asked me to show him the specific places I didn't like. He didn't say anything until I'd finished, and then he pointed out that my eyelids could be improved. And he was right.

'I wanted to set a date for the surgery immediately, but he refused. He told me to go home and think about it before we made an appointment for the operation.

'I was only in hospital overnight after the surgery, which was done under local anaesthesia.

'When I was leaving the hospital, the surgeon told me that I should try not to talk, laugh, or move around for a few days and that I should sleep on my back with lots of pillows. He also told me not to use my eyes, especially not to read or watch television. Fortunately, there are plenty of interesting radio programmes.

'After surgery the nurse surrounded my head with cotton wadding and then put a compression-type bandage over that. In the back of my neck there was a drain that led into the bandages. That was taken out after a couple of days.

'I didn't have any pain from the face lift, but there was some discomfort from the stitches. The surgeon said that I could take codeine for the problem, but not aspirin, because it can lead to bleeding.

'The day after the surgery I felt "spaced out", but not in any pain. I just lay in bed and didn't think about the operation. I was in bed at home for about a week. The restrictions on using my eyes lasted for several days, and then I was to use them only a bit each day.

'After ten days I could put on make up, and I bought some special make up to cover the scars.

'Two weeks later I made a lunch date with four women friends and débuted my face lift. I know some people feel reluctant to talk about cosmetic surgery, but I would have missed a terrific part of the experience if I hadn't shared it with my friends. One of them said I looked as I did when she first met me, and that had been ten years earlier. I looked like I'd had a wonderful rest.

'After five months I am still tender and numb where the cuts were made, and I'm tender behind the ears. At the back of the scalp, where the drain was, there's a knob of flesh; that takes a long time to go away. I have to remember to tell my hairdresser about it every time I have my hair done.

'I didn't tell my three daughters about the surgery. One is married and doesn't live near by, and two were away at university when I had the operation. When my daughters at university came home during their holidays, they were surprised and delighted. One of their friends came over to visit, and she said, "Mrs Wilson, your new hairstyle is terrific. You look wonderful."

'I think that after a face lift, you're more likely to be affected by things that are bad for your skin. If I have too much to drink at a party or have a sleepless night, I look worse than I would have looked before the surgery.

'All in all, I'm very glad I had it, and I'm very pleased with the results.'

It happens in everyone's life: one day you look in the mirror and see that your face is losing the battle with the force of gravity. Skin has loosened and begun to sag in the face and neck. Maybe there's also drooping of the upper eyelids, and bags under the eyes. Sometimes the experience of looking at this other you can be pretty depressing, because most of us continue to think of ourselves as we were when we were young. A London plastic surgeon comments, 'We used to say, "Grow old gracefully," because we didn't have anything else to offer. Now there is safe and effective surgery to get rid of sagging and loose skin and to turn the facial clock back five to ten years.'

Often you can tell simply by looking in the mirror whether a face lift would help. Or you might go through old family albums and find a picture of yourself five to ten years ago. Is the difference quite noticeable? (Of course, if you weren't happy with your looks when the picture was taken, you won't be any happier after a face lift, and the operation would be a waste of money.)

There are two simple tests you can do in front of a mirror to see if the surgery would help. For the first, place your palms against the sides of your face (middle finger at your hairline, jaws resting on your palms). Gently draw the skin back and up, but don't stretch your eyes or mouth. For the second test, place your fingers (pointed towards your back) along the sides of your neck (little fingers just touching the bottoms of the ears). Gently draw this skin back to see if you have loose skin on your neck. If during either of these tests you see significant improvement, you may want to consult a plastic surgeon about a face lift.

Although many people believe that a face lift is primarily for the upper face, the most dramatic changes produced by the operation are in the lower face, chin, and neck, thanks partly to improved techniques effected in the last several years.

If you'd like to postpone a face lift as long as possible, modifications in life-style can help. Avoid smoking and sunbathing. Smoking cuts the blood supply to the skin, and sun ages the skin prematurely. Be moderate in using alcohol. It would also be very nice if you could pick your parents: our genes play a significant role in the way our skin ages.

Throughout this discussion of face lifts, we are considering *full* face lifts and *not* the so-called mini-lift, or tuck. Responsible surgeons caution that the mini-lift is worthless. In a mini-lift the surgeon makes an incision in the lower temple area and removes a small amount of excess skin from the cheeks. The result is usually a temporary tightening of the cheek skin. One plastic surgeon says, 'You look fine for about fifteen days and then the effects disappear and you might as well not have had the surgery.' Another adds, 'A mini-lift lasts just about long enough for the surgeon to get your cheque deposited in the bank.'

A full face lift is another story, however, and can make a gratifying and long-lasting change in the appearance of your face and neck. As you consider the operation, you should realise that it is a long and major procedure in which the surgeon must be meticulously careful so that possible complications are avoided.

Consultation

With a face lift, surgeons want to be extra certain that your expectations are realistic—that you don't expect to look eighteen again. One plastic surgeon adds, 'The physician has to be sensitive to when patients are bothered by the signs of ageing, like the looseness of skin and the deep wrinkles. One woman in her forties may not be concerned by such signs as laxity of skin, whereas another woman in her forties may be suffering real pain from these signs of ageing.'

The surgeon will also explain whether a face lift will alter the features that are disturbing you. For example, if you are bothered by frown lines, forehead lines, or fine lines above the mouth, you should know that you won't find them gone *or even improved* after a face lift. Those involve other operations, as do the eyelids, both lower and upper. If you want other problems corrected at the same time as the face lift, both cost and length of the surgery will increase.

If you wish more than one correction, the surgeon may recommend (because of your general health or your financial resources) that you have the two operations done separately, at an interval of some months or a year. Usually he or she will want to correct first the problem that's bothering you most. As one says, 'I've had patients who are bothered more by baggy eyelids than by sagging skin. If that's the case, I suggest taking care of the eyelids first.'

During the consultation the surgeon may or may not show you before-and-after photographs of other patients. As noted earlier, there is controversy about whether that's wise, because such photos may lead to unrealistic expectations, given your skin type or your life-style. You may see the results of a face lift on a person with fair, dry skin and expect the same results for yourself—but, if you have dark, oily skin, you probably won't get them, because fair, dry skin tends to respond better to the surgery.

The surgeon will also want to be sure that you're at the correct weight for your body and are not planning to lose weight. In fact the loss of weight in middle age often prompts people to seek face lifts. When young people lose weight, the skin has enough elasticity to spring back into shape; in middle age, skin usually sags after weight loss. So the best time to have a face lift is *after* weight loss, not before.

Preferred Age

People often peg forty-five or fifty as the age at which one has a face lift. But there really is no single age that's the 'right' time, because everyone ages differently. A plastic surgeon explains, 'We all have different bone structures, different skin structures, different elasticity, different hormonal balances, different types of exposure to sun, cigarettes, alcohol, and that sort of thing. In people who've had their skin weathered by exposure to extreme sun and cigarette smoking, the skin's structural aspects won't be as good as those in light complexioned individuals who have really taken care of their skin through the years; such people obviously have better results in a face lift.'

There is no minimum or maximum age for a face lift. What's important is how you feel about your looks. With most people, signs of ageing in the face and neck become obvious some time between ages forty-five and fifty-five.

A plastic surgeon comments, 'Just as there's no rule on how early you can have a face lift, there's also no upper cut-off age for the operation. Today's society puts a tremendous stress on appearance at all points of the age spectrum. I've done a few women as young as forty-one and forty-two; in some other countries, such as America, women have face lifts while still in their thirties. The oldest person to whom I've given a face lift was eighty-four. Naturally I was extra cautious about operating on someone that age and insisted on a full testing and complete medical examination. She'd never been in

74

hospital before and had no major health problems, so I did the surgery; I used local anaesthetic because I felt it was less risky on someone that age.'

A 'juvenile' face lift is sometimes done on young people to help alleviate skin problems such as severe acne scarring.

Hospitalisation

Time spent in hospital will depend both on the type of anaesthetic used and on whether you're to undergo another procedure, such as eyelids or forehead, in addition to the face lift. In a few cases, patients have the surgery early in the morning and go home that evening; in others, the patient leaves twenty-four hours after the surgery. More usual is a period of two to three days in hospital. During the week following surgery you will usually have to visit the surgeon's consulting rooms once or twice to have dressings attended to.

Anaesthesia

Many surgeons prefer general anesthesia, though the operation can be done under local anaesthesia.

Procedure

Before the operation some surgeons shave off about an inch of hair along the line of the incision. Others merely part the hair along the incision line. Neither method should cause any appearance problem afterwards; if the hair is shaved, you should be able to comb your hair over the incision line. (If it's important to you whether the surgeon shaves or just parts the hair, put that item on your list of questions for the consultation.)

A plastic surgeon describes his method: 'I begin my incision in the scalp in the temporal area. Then I come down just in front of the ear, and I follow the ear around the lobe and into the concha [part of the external ear], then

75

on to the mastoid region [the bone behind the ear], and then into the posterior hairline. How high or low I go into the posterior hairline depends on the individual patient. If I need to get greater pull on the neck, I go low in the hairline. If the looseness is mainly in the cheeks and jowls, and I'm not so concerned with the neck, then I'll go higher in the hairline.

'I then separate the skin from the tissue beneath it [this is called undermining: if you have ever removed the skin from a chicken breast, you have an idea of the procedure]. The undermining is the key to the success of a face lift. I loosen the skin totally from the temple to the outer end of the eyebrow, over the cheeks, and halfway down the neck. I raise the skin flap and expose the tissue underneath. If there's laxness in the muscle tissue, I can make it more firm with stitches. Next, I draw the skin back and up, trim off the excess, and suture the skin into its new place. 'I also put a drain in, underneath the neck area and exiting in the mastoid area behind the neck in the hairline. The drain is removed on the second day after the operation.'

It's important that the surgeon pulls back just enough skin—not too little and not too much. If too little is pulled back, the operation won't achieve the desired result; if too much, your face will have a stretched, perhaps startled, look—and there can be medical complications.

The face lift alone will take about three hours—longer if you're having another procedure done at the same time, such as eyelids or forehead.

There is no difference in the face-lift procedure for black skin, though it generally begins to wrinkle later in life than white skin does.

Men considering face-lift surgery should know that sideburns can be greatly diminished by the procedure: someone who's cultivating a handsome set of sideburns and wants to keep them should tell the surgeon at the consultation. The technique for the operation can be changed slightly to preserve the sideburns without affecting the result of the face lift. Men will also find that, because skin is pulled back and up in the operation, some of their hairbearing skin will end up just behind their ears. They will either have to shave it or undergo electrolysis to have it permanently removed.

Aftermath

After the surgery you'll probably be encased in a compression dressing around the head, including neck and cheeks. The dressing is designed to prevent bleeding and minimise swelling by keeping the tissues in place. Some surgeons bandage the eyes; others don't, because they fear frightening patients. (If you would be very upset or frightened at having your eyes bandaged, check with the surgeon at the consultation to be sure it won't be done.) The dressing stays on for twenty-four to thirty-six hours; after that you may require a lighter dressing, or none at all.

Usually the surgeon will have ice packs applied to your face regularly for the first twenty-four hours in hospital and will have you continue to do the same for several days at home in order to help reduce the swelling. The amount of swelling varies with the individual; there may be a little, or there may be a lot. In either case it usually disappears within two weeks.

For the first twenty-four hours you probably won't be allowed solid foods. After that you'll gradually build up to soft food and then to a normal diet by the end of a week. This prevents overuse of the facial muscles in eating.

Surgeons and patients agree that there is little pain associated with a properly done face lift; but there can be discomfort, especially from the dressings that you'll have to wear during the day or two after surgery.

Convalescence

During your convalescence at home, don't invite over your wittiest friends. If you do, ask them to avoid telling you jokes. During the first days after surgery you should laugh and talk as little as possible. Again, this precaution avoids overuse of the facial muscles.

77

The stitches in front of the ear begin coming out after five days. Usually, all the stitches are out by the twelfth day.

Most surgeons agree that you should plan to be off work for two to three weeks, so that the swelling can clear up completely. You may need less time, but this cannot be predicted.

During your convalescence you won't be able to do any strenuous exercises or lifting. You'll also be advised to sleep on your back with several pillows under your head.

For about a week you won't be able to wash your hair, and then you'll wash it with a gingerly touch to avoid disturbing the stitches.

With women, your skin type and the rate at which you're healing will determine when you can wear make up: ask the surgeon just before you leave the hospital. Men will want to ask the surgeon how soon they can shave safely. Usually you can use an electric razor earlier than a standard razor; with either, it's important to avoid pressure that could pull the skin.

Scars

Naturally, such extensive incisions involve scarring. But except for the scar in front of the ear, the scars are hidden in your hair. The scars in front of your ears should fade in about three months.

Complications

One reason that face-lift surgery takes so long is that a number of problems can develop. Most common is a haematoma (a collection of blood under the skin). The scars may also be a complication; some people simply heal better than others.

Very rarely, the skin is pulled too tight and a condition known as necrosis develops. When this occurs, the skin around the incision dies and sloughs off.

With most face lifts there is decreased sensation, or

numbness, for a time, as Christine MacKay reported. It often clears up within a few weeks; sometimes it takes several months. In a few cases the partial numbness is permanent.

Finally, the surgeon is working very near the five branches of the facial nerve, and there is the possibility of damage to them. If the facial nerve is injured but not cut, the result is a temporary paralysis that lasts for several days. If the nerve is cut during surgery, the surgeon can stitch the severed nerve together. Movement and feeling should return after several weeks.

The most significant problem occurs if there is injury to a nerve that controls forehead muscles, resulting in an inability to wrinkle one side of the forehead. Usually, in time the function returns. If not, the surgeon must decide whether to operate a second time and try to stitch together the ends of the cut nerves (an attempt that is frequently unsuccessful) or, rather, to cut the same nerve branch on the other side so that the forehead won't wrinkle at all. As one surgeon says, 'At least that way its symmetrical.'

Durability of Result

Estimates of how long a face lift lasts do vary, because, as mentioned above, a number of factors can influence the rate at which your face will age. Some surgeons say that a face lift usually lasts about five years; others say it may last ten to fifteen years. Usually men's face lifts last longer than women's, because the top layer of a man's skin is thicker than a woman's.

There's no limit to the number of face lifts you can have to help maintain a fresh appearance. However, a second or third face lift won't make you look as you did after the first one: each face lift turns the clock back, but it can't stop the ageing process.

Though some gossip columnists—and some unscrupulous practitioners—make face lifts sound as common and simple as manicures, they are major surgery and can end in unpleasant complications. But properly done by a responsible plastic surgeon, a face lift can raise your spirits and morale.

10 Eyelid and Eyebag Lifts

Time is a dressmaker specialising in alterations.—Faith Baldwin

Ted Stevens of Richmond, Surrey, is fifty and an executive with a London hotel group. He had surgery on his upper and lower eyelids.

'I became conscious of the bags under my eyes about two years ago. It wasn't until perhaps a year later that I noticed my upper eyelids were drooping as well.

'Whenever I thought about it—sometimes when I looked in the mirror while I was shaving—I was bothered. I'd say to myself, 'Ted, you're looking old.' But I'd put it out of my mind. After all, I had a lovely family, an interesting well-paid job, and good friends. And physically I felt as I did when I was twenty-five.

'Then I was invited as a representative of our hotel group on a trip to France with some other people in the travel business. My wife came along, and I expected to nave a wonderful time.

'The first day we had a meeting in the morning and then lunch at Brasserie Lipp in Paris. Those of us who were there for the business trip were scheduled for an afternoon meeting. As we were leaving the restaurant, my boss said, 'Ted, you look tired. Maybe you'd rather a nap than a meeting.' I said I felt fine—which I did—and went along with him.

'After the business trip ended a few days later, my wife and I stayed in Paris to visit a couple we hadn't seen for several years.

'We had a wonderful time that afternoon, roaming all around the Left Bank. Early in the evening we stopped at a café, and my friend George said to me, 'Do you think we should cancel our evening plans? You look exhausted.'

'I said I wasn't any more tired than anyone else, and I was very much looking forward to going to dinner and a nightclub as we'd planned.

'When my wife and I went back to our hotel room to dress, I looked at myself in the mirror, and I knew he was right. I looked as though I hadn't slept for weeks.

'When we got home to London, I asked my wife what she thought about my appearance. She hemmed and hawed a bit—told me I worked very hard and had a good deal of responsibility—but finally she admitted that I did look tired.

'It took me six more weeks to work up the courage to ask her if she'd agree that I could spend some of our savings for an operation on my eyelids and eye bags. I went to lengths to assure her that I was very happy with my marriage and family, but I was sick of looking like a tired sixty-five rather than a relatively fit fifty—which I am. She agreed that I could spend the money.

'Our GP is about ten or twelve years younger than I am. I was a little reluctant to ask him for the name of a plastic surgeon, but there didn't seem any other course. He was matter-of-fact about it, said he understood the problem, and referred me to a plastic surgeon in central London.

'The surgeon asked me some questions about why I wanted to look younger. He must have been satisfied with the answers, because he agreed to do the surgery.

'He said I should take a week off my job, because I'd have to rest at home after the surgery, but he also said I would be operated on with local anaesthetic early in the morning at a private hospital and could go home late in the afternoon.

'After the surgery there was some swelling and bruising around my eyes, but it wasn't bad. I was apprehensive that the surgeon would bandage my eyes, but he didn't. For the first day after the surgery, my wife applied ice around my eyes, and I stayed in bed for forty-eight hours, as instructed.

'To tell the truth, I felt wonderful. I made my wife call the surgeon the day after the operation and ask if we could go for a drive in the country as long as she drove the car. As you can guess, he said, 'No, no, no.'

'After the stitches came out about five days later and the bruising disappeared, I took a long look in the mirror. I don't look as young as I feel, but for the first time in years, I don't look older than I am.'

What causes the drooping eyelids and the eye bags that can suggest drowsiness and make us look years older than we are? When they appear in young people in their late teens or early twenties, they're usually hereditary. When they appear in middle-aged and older people, a plastic surgeon explains, 'it's very much like the sagging of other skin on your face—that is, the law of gravity finally wins. But sagging around the eyes may start earlier than sagging of other skin, often at about thirty-five, because the skin around the eyes is thinner than other skin on the face; in fact it's the thinnest skin on the whole body. It's also looser. And if it's been exposed to too much sun, alcohol, or cigarettes, that will show.

'When you think of the work your eyelids have to do, it's not surprising that there's drooping. You blink every four to five seconds. As you age, there's excess skin around the eyes, and the lid has to support the additional weight each time you blink. It can't snap back, because the skin isn't as elastic as it was when you were younger; instead it droops.

'The operation to correct drooping eyelids and eye bags is called blepharoplasty. With the upper lid, it's designed to remove any skin pleat that can come down almost as a hood, usually in the outer third of the eye, and get rid of puffiness in the inner part of the upper lid. With the lower lid, the surgery corrects the bag and the very gross pleating of the lid. Bags under the eyes are usually caused by fat. The fat itself is normal, because the eyeball rests in a bony cavity and the globe is encircled by a sort of shock-absorber of fat. That fat is normal and is supposed to stay where it belongs. However, sometimes it protrudes forward because the fibrous sheet that's designed to keep it back is weak. It's hereditarily weak in certain families.

'Some people develop vision problems. If the ptosis [drooping of the eyelids] is severe, the skin can hang over so much that it obstructs the vision. If that problem is coupled with puffiness under the eyes, which can force the lower lids upwards, you have a narrowing of the eyes. Or excess skin around the outer canthus [outer corner of the eye] can interfere with peripheral vision. If in fact there is interference with vision, the surgery can be done on NHS.

'Very often, blepharoplasty is done in conjunction with a face lift. But it doesn't have to be. And the patient might not have surgery on both upper and lower lids; he or she may need only one of those procedures.

'This surgery does not correct chronic dark circles under the eyes—there is no surgery to correct that condition. We find these 'shiners' most often in people with allergic tendancies who may have asthma, hay fever, and so on. The dark circles do not represent a lack of sleep, but a very local, mild congestion of the veins in that area, which drain into the nasal sinuses. Treating the allergy, usually with antihistamines, will often help that condition.'

Consultation

As usual, surgeons want to be sure that your motives are sound and your expectations realistic. They also want to be certain that the cause of puffiness around the eyes is indeed fat and not swelling—an accumulation of fluid that may be caused by sinus, allergy, kidney, or thyroid problems. If the puffiness is due to swelling rather than fat deposits, the cause must be diagnosed and then treated.

It's important to know what the operation can't do as well as what it can. As noted, it won't clear up chronic dark circles; it won't take care of any problems in the cheek area below the eyelid; and it won't eliminate so-called crow's-feet, lines at the outer corners of the eyes.

Some people over forty, the usual candidates for eyelid surgery, may also suffer from glaucoma. If the condition is controlled by medication, it is no barrier to having cosmetic surgery on the eyelids. If you know you have glaucoma, be sure to tell the surgeon during the consultation, so that he or she will have information about your glaucoma medication when prescribing drugs to be used during or after the operation.

Hospitalisation

The hospital stay can vary, depending on your age and general health. Fortunately, the skin around the eyes heals very quickly. In some cases you won't even have to stay in hospital overnight; in others you may remain one night or sometimes two. (Length of hospital stay will also depend on whether you're having another procedure as well as the eyelid surgery.)

Anaesthesia

If you're having just eyelid surgery, the surgeon may well use a local anaesthetic (with sedation such as intravenous Valium). If you're having this surgery in conjunction with another procedure, such as a face lift, you and the surgeon may prefer a general anaesthetic.

Procedure

Sometime before the surgery, the face and hair are cleaned with an antispetic solution.

A plastic surgeon describes his procedure: 'For the upper lid, I make the incision in the fold of the lid and extend it just beyond the outer borders of the lid, ending with an upward curve. What I'm usually doing in this operation is shortening the muscle that elevates the lid.

'Work on the lower lids is more difficult and intricate; it takes the bulk of my time and concentration during the surgery. I make the incision close to the border of the lid and again extend it slightly beyond the outer borders of the lid, finishing off with a downward curve. I then remove the fatty tissue and any excess skin and suture the incision closed.'

85

After the stitching, some surgeons apply antibiotic ointment to the area.

The operation for both drooping eyelids and eye bags takes a total of one and a half to two hours for both eyes.

Aftermath

There is disagreement among surgeons about whether the eyes should be bandaged after the surgery. One plastic surgeon says, 'I don't bandage; I think it's much better for you to be able to take the ice compresses off and look around so you know that you haven't been blinded. Those who bandage feel that mild pressure keeps the swelling at a minimum. I haven't found that it does.'

For the first twenty-four hours or so, you should keep applying ice compresses to the area around your eyes to help control swelling. You will also be advised to keep your head elevated.

In the first day or two after surgery, some patients experience double vision, but that disappears within forty-eight hours.

For the first few days after surgery, you'll have difficulty moving your eyelids.

There will be some bruising and swelling around the eyes, but both conditions should clear up in one to two weeks.

The stitches come out from three days to one week after the surgery.

Convalescence

For eyelid surgery alone, you need take only one week off work (though many surgeons would prefer that you make it two weeks). In some cases, if it's very important to you, you can go back earlier than that. The bruising and stitches can be disguised quite well with sunglasses. If you're keeping the nature of the surgery a secret, one surgeon says, 'the best white lie is to tell people you had eyelid cysts removed.'

One surgeon describes a small postsurgical problem

and its solution. 'The eyes may look very good, but they will still look a little stiff and a little 'starey' for about two to three months, and I tell patients this before the surgery. It isn't bad, but the expression will be a little tense rather than soft, and the lids will feel tight for at least three weeks. For this condition I give patients exercises of the lids to do during their convalescence. I have them squeeze the lids together as tightly as they can—ten times a row in a series and ten series a day—and it's very helpful in getting rid of the oedema [swelling caused by fluid]. If there has been upper-lid surgery, I have them gently stroke the incision from the nose outwards with their fingers using a little moisturising cream. That's a mini-massage and also helps to get rid of swelling.'

Since surgeons want you to keep your blood pressure low while healing, you'll also be advised to avoid strenuous exercise such as lifting and to avoid bending for the first five to seven days.

After about two weeks the use of eye make up and contact lenses can be resumed.

For some months after the surgery, sunbathing isn't permitted.

Scars

The skin around the eyes heals very well, so that when the scars fade, they should be virtually undetectable. The upper lid incision is hidden in the natural fold of the lid, and the lower-lid incision is close to the border of the lid.

Complications

Complications are rare, but when they occur, it's often because the surgeon hasn't removed exactly the right amount of skin.

If too little skin has been taken away, the improvement won't be as significant as it should be.

A more serious problem occurs if the surgeon removes too much skin. Then the eye can't be closed, even for sleeping; as a result, often the cornea becomes dry and irritated, and the function of the eyelid in protecting the eye from dust, grime, and other assaults from the outside world is thwarted. A surgeon who has treated patients of other plastic surgeons has seen this complication only twice in his thirty years of practice. 'It's about as likely as that the ceiling of the operating theatre will fall in and kill both the patient and me. On the two occasions that I've treated it, I had the patients do the same exercises as I give patients after normal surgery [see 'Convalescence', above] but I have them do more series each day. And I have them use a small, thin strip of paper tape to push the lower eyelid upwards. There you are pressing the eyelids into their proper position. In extremely rare cases—I've only heard about one—it's necessary to use a small skin graft. Such a graft would not be noticeable, because the skin around the eyes heals so well.'

A minor complication is that the eyes tear too copiously or too little, which means that they aren't getting the proper lubrication. The problem usually solves itself spontaneously, but there are drops available to treat both conditions.

You could also develop tiny pimples in the area around the stitches. If that happens, call your surgeon, because they'll have to be pierced with a sterile needle.

The most horrifying possible complication is explained by an ophthalmologist: 'It's extremely rare, but you can get a disastrous haemorrhage behind the eye, and you can lose the vision. There are, to my knowledge, at least twenty to forty cases in the world [medical] literature of people who have gone blind in one eye after having this operation. Although the risk in percentage terms is very small, it's not frightfully amusing if your number comes up.'

Durability of Results

The correction for drooping upper lids lasts ten to fifteen years. The results of eye-bag surgery last at least that long, and often longer.

Plastic surgeons consider eyelid and eye-bag surgery among the safest surgical procedures in their repertoire. And they agree that, for the patient, no other cosmetic operation provides such a swift change in appearance.

11 Other Facial Surgery

Then Sir Launcelot saw her visage,
but he wept not greatly, but sighed.
—Sir Thomas Malory

A major facial operation, such as nose alteration or face lift, is often supplemented by one or more of four other procedures.

Chin Implant

Chin implants are often done in conjunction with nose alterations to give a pleasingly balanced profile. Surgeons estimate that about ninety per cent of patients who want nose alterations also need a chin implant. Of course, the implant can be done by itself to correct a receding chin.

The incision can be made through the mouth in front of the gums, or it can be made just under the chin. The surgeon then creates a pocket, into which he or she puts either cartilage from the patient's own body, or an implant of silicone. A plastic surgeon says that when he does the chin implant in connection with nose surgery, he uses cartilage from the nose. 'I think the silicone implant tends to make the patient look too "jaw-ey"; I prefer to use the patient's own tissue.'

The opening is then stitched closed, and a bandage is placed around the chin to prevent movement of the implant. The dressing is removed within three or four days.

The chin implant takes about half an hour to perform. There is bruising, which will last for ten days to two weeks. Patients will also be on a soft-food diet for a week to ten days to minimise movement of the mouth.

There are two possible complications: infections, if the implant isn't from your own tissue; and incorrect positioning of the implant.

Double-chin Removal

Removal of the fat that causes a double chin can be done as a separate operation or, as is very often the case, in conjunction with a face lift.

The surgeon makes an incision about one and a half inches long just under and behind the chin. Then excess fat and skin are removed and the skin is stitched together. The scar heals as a fine line and, because of its location, is not visible.

Forehead Lift

A forehead lift attempts to eliminate or reduce deep horizontal lines on the forehead caused by worry, age, or habitual puckering of the eyebrows.

A plastic surgeon says, 'The forehead lift is sometimes done at the same time as a face lift. For the operation I make a coroneal incision—that is, I cut from ear to ear about one inch behind the hairline. Then I separate the skin from the subcutaneous tissue, taking care to preserve the nerves. I remove the excess skin and subcutaneous tissue and suture the wound.

'To make the surgery effective and the result natural-looking, the patient must have a low hairline, because the hairline after the surgery is moved up at least three-quarters of an inch.

91

'I use a pressure-type dressing, which the patient wears for about a week. There will be bruising, sometimes severe, around the forehead and upper eyes for up to two weeks after the surgery. The sutures are removed after seven to ten days.

'The two possible complications are damage to the nerves, and hair loss caused by the tension when the forehead skin and scalp skin are brought together.'

Note: Many surgeons do not think this surgery effects sufficient change or produces sufficiently long-lasting results to justify the operation.

Eyebrow Lift

For those whose eyebrows have drooped with the passage of time, there is the eyebrow lift, often done in connection with surgery for eyelids and eye bags.

Surgeons can make an incision just above the hairline of the eyebrow, remove some skin, and pull the eyebrow up. In many cases this has the additional positive effect of raising the upper eyelid.

People who have a good deal of eyebrow hair find that it usually hides the surgical scar. Others get a prominent scar. Women can usually hide such a scar with make up.

12 Chemical Skin Peel

Beauty is but a flower
Which wrinkles will devour ...
    —Thomas Nashe

Catherine Dodge, who lives in Bristol, is fifty-five and married to an industrial engineer. When she made an appointment with a cosmetic plastic surgeon, she knew that she didn't like the appearance of her facial skin, but she wasn't sure what could be done about it.

'The surgeon told me that the laxity of my facial skin could be helped by a face lift, but that the fine lines above and below my mouth and between my eyebrows would remain. For these he recommended a chemical skin peel, to be done at the same time as the face lift. He said that my fair skin should give good results.

'When I approached my husband, I told him that I was going to have a skin cancer removed from my chest—which was true—and that I wanted to have some cosmetic surgery done at the same time. He must have been in a good mood, because he agreed.

'The tests that are done before an operation were done on an outpatient basis, and I went into hospital on the morning of the surgery. I was in hospital for about three days. All three procedures—the removal of the skin cancer, the face lift, and the skin peel—were done at the same time.

'I didn't sleep for the whole night after the surgery. But I was in no great pain except for a splitting headache, for which I was given a non-aspirin painkiller. I had bandages from the face lift, and tape in the areas where the

93

surgeon had done the skin peel. I had ice packs on constantly to reduce the swelling. There was a vague sensation of stinging in the chin where I'd had the skin peel.

'The tape caused some discomfort. I could feel the edges of the tape drawing away from my skin, and that hurt. Two days later, when the surgeon came in to take the tape off, I asked for a painkiller. He gave me a shot, but I was very sick to my stomach after the tape was removed. He later told me that it was probably from the medication and was an unusual reaction.

'After he took the tape off, the surgeon sprinkled a mustard-yellow powder where the tape had been. For two days at home, the area had to be kept covered with powder. Three days after he removed the tape, I went to his consulting room, and he gave me instructions about using Crisco several times a day on my face. The skin started coming off with the Crisco about five days after I started using it, and I kept using the Crisco until the skin was smooth a few weeks later.

'There was swelling in the area where I had the peel, and that lasted for a month. My skin was bright pink, as though it had been sunburned. I also had a great deal of itching afterwards, but you're not allowed to scratch; you can just press the spot that itches. I used some anti-itching pills and creams. I also wore white gloves when I slept so that I wouldn't accidentally scratch my face. The surgeon told me that I had to stay out of the sun for six months, which I did. If I even went on errands on a sunny day, I always wore a hat with a brim.

'I've had some permanent pigmentation changes, so I have to use two different kinds of make up on my face.

'Actually, I'm thinking of having some more chemical peeling done for some other fine wrinkles, but my husband wants me to wait for a while. I think he hopes I'll forget. He's never directly said anything about it, but I don't think he likes the sound of what they do to you, and he knows how awful I looked in those days at home after the surgery.'

One of the bothersome signs of ageing is the appearance of fine lines around the mouth and at the cheeks, crow's-feet around the eyes, and/or forehead lines. Often these wrinkles can be removed by a process called chemical skin peeling. It is not, as some people think, an alternative to a face lift. A face lift treats the laxity of the skin; a chemical skin peel affects the texture of the skin.

Because a dangerous compound is used, chemical skin peeling must be considered with *great caution*. Candidates for the procedure should be screened for susceptibility to organ damage; and—even given careful screening—there is a risk of terrible damage if the process is done by someone who isn't properly trained.

The skin consists of three levels: the top layers are the epidermis, next is the dermis, and under that is fat. With a chemical skin peel, a solution made up of phenol (carbolic acid) and other components is painted on the skin and induces a second-degree burn that removes the epidermis and the upper layers of the dermis. The face swells; after the swelling goes down, a crust forms on the skin. When the crust comes off, there is new, smooth skin. Only the facial skin responds well to a chemical skin peel; there is too much danger of scarring in other areas.

Although you should search for a competent surgeon for any cosmetic procedure, it is vital that you have an experienced and responsible surgeon for a chemical skin peel. Otherwise you are running unreasonable risks of facial scarring and damage to the kidneys and brain.

Consultation

In your assessment of the surgeon, be sure to ask how many chemical skin peels he or she has done lately and what complications, if any, patients have experienced.

At the same time, the surgeon will be deciding whether you are a suitable patient. The plastic surgeon who operated on Catherine Dodge says, 'First the surgeon will consider your colouring and skin type. A chemical skin peel is not for people with dark, oily skin, because the peel can leave a halo on the skin, marking the edges of the treated area. It "takes" better on people with light complexions. I prefer a patient with blonde or red hair, blue eyes, and fair skin.

'If I'm not sure about the reaction of a patient's skin to the phenol solution, I do a test in front of or behind the ear near the hairline. If the results are good, which I'll know a few weeks after the test, I'll go ahead with the procedure.

'A partial chemical skin peel in the perioral area [the area around the mouth] can be done in conjunction with a face lift. I would not, however, do a full facial skin peel, which involves everything from the forehead to the jawline, in conjunction with a face lift, because that would compromise the blood supply.

'Sometimes I do a full chemical skin peel, if the patient needs it, as early as eight to ten weeks after the face lift. Sometimes I do a peel first, let several months go by, and then do the face lift. The full chemical peel will improve or eliminate the deep wrinkles and improve the appearance of the skin, but by itself it will do nothing for the laxity of the skin—the jowls, the fullness, the turkey-gobbler neck, the deep nasal-labial fold.

'At the consultation I also want to be very sure that the patient has no physical condition that would be adversely affected by the phenol [a major component, with toxic qualities, of the compound used in the skin peel]. A skin peel shouldn't be done on anyone with kidney disease, liver disease, heart disease, diabetes, or a tendency to keloids [raised scars]. Often, even if I have a complete medical history and it shows no evidence of kidney problems, I still have the patient's urine tested to be sure the kidneys are healthy.

'I also tell the patient she won't be able to go out for about ten days after the skin peel, in case she would need to make arrangements to have shopping and other errands taken care of by someone else.'

Chemical skin peels are not often done on NHS.

Hospitalisation

For a full facial skin peel, the usual time in hospital is three days. A peel on a small area of the face that is not done in conjunction with another procedure can sometimes be done on an outpatient basis.

Anaesthesia

If the skin peel is done by itself (and not in conjunction with another procedure, such as a face lift), surgeons often use only sedation, because elements in the solution act as a local anaesthetic.

Procedure

Your skin will be scrubbed with surgical soap and then cleansed again with ether, which draws out any remaining soap and also the oil normal in skin glands.

The nostrils are plugged so that you don't inhale the phenol fumes.

The liquid phenol solution is painted on the skin with cotton applicators, the depth of the burn controlled by the amount of solution the surgeon applies. Depending on the depth of the wrinkles, the surgeon will or will not apply adhesive tapes over the area that has been painted: the tapes prolong the phenol's action and deepen its penetration. The tape is applied in small strips; with a full skin peel, openings are left for eyes, nostrils, and mouth.

A full facial chemical skin peel takes about thirty minutes to perform.

Aftermath

Six or seven hours after the peel, your face will begin to swell; some patients' eyes swell shut. Ice packs are used to keep the swelling down.

If your skin has been taped, the 'mask' will be left on for forty-eight hours. During that time you'll stay in bed with your head elevated. You will be asked to talk and move your face as little as possible. And you'll be on a liquid diet, fed through a straw.

Surgeons say that patients are usually uncomfortable for the first twenty-four to forty-eight hours but rarely have complaints after that.

A plastic surgeon describes the next steps: 'After the first day the patient will notice a fluid seeping through the mask. I take the tape off a day later. That can hurt, and most patients have a painkiller to get through the experience.

'When the tape is off, I put on a thymol iodide powder. Within twenty-four hours it adheres to the skin and forms a crust. The patient should apply more of this powder at home, three times a day.'

Convalescence

A plastic surgeon describes the recovery period: 'About five to seven days later, I have patients apply Crisco to promote the crust's falling off. Some surgeons prefer Vaseline, but I find that many patients break out from it; and some use other ointments. I caution the patients to be *very* careful not to remove the crust that remains. I know it's hard to keep from picking at scabs, but it's absolutely essential that the patient does not pull in any way at the crusted area; if you do, you can be left with scarring. After about seven to ten days of the Crisco treatment, the scabs fall off.

'When the crust comes off, the skin has no wrinkles— partly because it's still swollen. I warn patients that when the swelling goes down, some lines will reappear.

'The skin will be very red for about one to three weeks after the crust comes off, and it will have a grainy texture. Usually, women can resume wearing cosmetics about a fortnight after the crust comes off. There will be some pigmentation changes that will have to be masked with make up. Those changes may last for as long as six months; sometimes the changes are permanent, but not usually. After a month the skin's texture returns to normal.

'Another strong caution I give my patients is that they *must not* expose the skin to the sun for at least six months. If there's any chance that they will be in sunlight, they should wear a hat with a wide brim and apply a sun block.'

Complications

Possible complications from chemical skin peels include prolonged redness of the skin, permanent change in pigmentation (as Catherine Dodge experienced), increased sensitivity of the skin to sunlight, and the formation of raised scars. Sometimes little whitehead pimples form, but they usually disappear within a few weeks.

A major complication can occur if the person performing the procedure makes an error and allows too much phenol to enter the bloodstream too rapidly. In such a case, vital organs can be affected and even destroyed.

If you are contemplating a chemical skin peel—especially a full facial peel—you should think long and hard, balancing the problem your facial wrinkles cause you against the risks involved. One plastic surgeon, who won't do chemical skin peels, said, 'I'd really like to see more data on the effects of the chemical used in skin peels on the different organs. I'm not saying that the results would be bad, but I would like to know what they are before I agreed to do the procedure.' When asked why he would not perform chemical skin peels, another surgeon said, 'I'm a surgeon. I heal people; I don't burn them.'

13 Dermabrasion

You don't have to suffer to be a poet.
Adolescence is enough suffering for anyone.
—John Ciardi

Fulham resident Ross Hughes, twenty-six and single, is a freelance writer who specialises in articles about rock music. Four years ago he underwent dermabrasion for the removal of acne scars.

'I'm not a good advert for dermabrasion, because I wasn't happy with the results. But I have to say that my unhappiness was my own fault—I expected far too much.

'As I see it, my current occupation is a direct result of my having had acne. I spent most of my teenage years in my bedroom listening to rock music. I had very bad acne—my face was just a mass of red spots—and I could hardly bear to go to school. When school was over for the day, I'd go home as fast as I could and hole up in my room. I was the opposite of the kid who gives his parents worry because he's out all night or spends too much time away from home. My parents worried because I never went anywhere and had only a few friends. Most of them looked almost as bad as I did.

'About the time I was twenty-one, the acne itself cleared up. But I was left with great scars on my face. If you'd photographed a section of my face and put it next to a photograph of a section of the moon and its craters, you'd have been hard put to tell the difference.

'Around the same time, a magazine accepted an article I wrote about a rock group. While I was looking through another magazine directed to teenagers and young adults,

I saw a piece about dermabrasion. I was fascinated. I knew it would be the answer for me.

'I got the name of a plastic surgeon through some contacts I'd made in the rock music field. I went to see him, and he agreed there was a problem. He said, "Would you be happy with a forty to fifty per cent improvement?" I said yes, which was a lie, because I was somehow sure that for me it would be one hundred per cent improvement.

'I sold my motorcycle to pay for the treatments. I asked that they be done under general anaesthetic, because I don't really like the sight of blood.

'I had a bandage on for the first day; I looked just awful when it was taken off. I thought, This is what I sold my motorcycle for?

'But after the crusts fell off, my face was very smooth, and rather pink. The surgeon warned me that it wouldn't stay that smooth or that pink, but I don't think I heard him. For the first time since I was thirteen, I had smooth skin!

'Once the swelling went down, the skin showed some evidence of the acne scars again. I was very disappointed, but I had exactly what the surgeon said I'd get—forty to fifty per cent improvement.

'The surgeon suggested that I would need two or three treatments, but I haven't had any after the first one.

'Instead I resorted to a solution that's been available to me all along: I've grown a full beard, and that has covered most of the pits.'

Many cosmetic surgery procedures are designed to counteract the effects of ageing, but dermabrasion is most often the resort of those who have suffered one of the age-old banes of adolescence—acne.

Fortunately, the use of antibiotics and other chemical remedies has revolutionised the treatment of acne in recent years. There are, however, those who suffer scars after the acne itself has died out or been controlled. In some cases those scars can be smoothed out by dermabrasion.

Dermabrasion has the same aim as chemical skin

101

peeling—the surgical destruction of the top layer of skin in the hope that the layers under it will heal more smoothly. Dermabrasion removes the top layer immediately, while chemical skin peeling leaves that layer in place while new skin forms under it. Chemical skin peeling is the more effective procedure to smooth fine wrinkles; dermabrasion is the better technique to provide relief for certain acne scars (and for similar scars, most commonly produced by chicken pox), to remove freckles, and to complete scar revision (see the chapter on that procedure). It can also help lessen fine lines and shallow wrinkles. Facial skin responds best to dermabrading, and in fact the technique isn't used on other parts of the body.

A plastic surgeon says, 'You'll find rather few plastic surgeons who dermabrade, because for many people—alas, often those with the most dramatic scarring—it's not a very good operation. I do dermabrasion because, for most of the patients with acne scars, there's nothing else to offer, and you do get significant improvement in selected cases. At a medical meeting in Toronto in 1979, a panel dealt with the amelioration of acne scars by aesthetic surgery, and it was generally agreed that it's an unsolved problem.

'The patients do generally feel somewhat better about themselves. If I didn't have the majority of them feeling reasonably happy, there'd be no point in doing it.'

When people are left with bad facial scars after an accident, perhaps having cut the face on a shattered windscreen, from six months to a year later they may have plastic surgery aimed at removing (or 'revising', as surgeons say) as many aspects of the scarring as possible. After such revision surgery, many surgeons routinely dermabrade the skin. A plastic surgeon comments, 'I'm not very enthusiastic about dermabrasion for scars. Many surgeons think that the final step in scar revision is dermabrasion, to smooth the edges a little bit. It certainly does no harm, but I think in most cases it doesn't do much good. Sometimes, if you have a scar that's rather like an acne scar, you may be able to smooth it out. Or you may have a very sharp line of skin tones—perhaps after a superficial burn has left a pale patch ringed by slightly darker pigmentation; occasionally dermabrasion can help that.'

Consultation

If you're considering dermabrasion for the usual reason— to have acne scars removed—the plastic surgeon will be concerned about the nature of the acne scars, whether the acne is under control, and what you expect of the procedure. The surgeon will carefully assess the type of acne scars you have, since only certain kinds benefit from dermabrasion. If you have deep ice-pick scars—small openings, but deep—you're not likely to get a good result. The acne scars that can be helped most are those that may be likened to moon craters; they have a sharp edge that casts a shadow, and a wide pit. The surgeon may be able to make an undulating edge, which catches the light less and is definitely an improvement over the sharp edges.

Surgeons doing dermabrasion are cautious to see that their prospective patients' expectations are realistic. Most emphasise that dermabrasion is a palliative, not a cure. The scars are not eliminated; they are simply made less noticeable. One surgeon says, 'If they think the surgeon is really going to clear up their skin, then they're hopeless as patients. I tell them honestly to put it on a scale of one to ten, with ten being the restoration of basically unscarred skin. If they would not be interested in an improvement at two or three on the scale, then I won't do it. I warn them that I'm not expecting much.'

Other plastic surgeons say that this view is unduly pessimistic: that the results of dermabrasion are generally satisfactory and there is often a fifty per cent improvement in the appearance of the skin.

Plastic surgeons also warn patients about possible pigment changes after dermabrasion. Says one, 'Ninety per cent of my patients are women, and most would accept a fairly striking colour change in return for smoothness, because make up can't cover irregularities in skin texture. However, if after dermabrasion the colour is a bit paler or darker—usually it's paler—they don't find that any great problem. But I want to be sure they're aware an alteration in skin colour is possible.'

Because the scars must be the right type and because some patients have unrealistic expectations of success, one surgeon estimates that one third to one half of the people who come for a consultation about dermabrasion do not proceed to surgery, whereas ninety to ninety-five per cent of all candidates for other cosmetic surgery who are accepted for the procedure do elect to have it.

When the dermabrasion is to involve an extensive area of the face, most surgeons test by doing a small patch first. If after a couple of months the results are clearly good and there is not much pigment change, the full dermabrasion can be done. If the results are less certain, a longer wait may be involved. The test not only tells the surgeon the effects of dermabrasion on your skin; it also tells *you* what's involved in the process.

A plastic surgeon says that in some cases he recommends a procedure other than dermabrasion for acne scars. 'Occasionally, one or two very big pits can actually be excised [cut out] surgically and closed with a fine (hairline) scar. That's better than dermabrasion. If you have really bad old acne scars whose pegs go down almost to the underlying muscle, I often recommend a juvenile face lift, in which I undermine the scars so they're detached from their underpeggings. When I pull the skin, they will slide a little way, which will very often help. I've had patients as young as twenty-three have this procedure.'

In many cases, dermabrasion can be done on NHS.

Preferred Age

The age of the patient is secondary to the state of the acne—whether it has disappeared or is under control. Surgeons differ about whether it's advisable to dermabrade while acne is still active. One refuses to consider it because he believes it can cause an acne flare-up. 'I wait until it's burnt out—and still get a flare-up sometimes.' A second, who thinks that in some cases dermabrasion actually helps to overcome acne, often will dermabrade while the acne is active. A third says, 'The acne should be pretty well under control before dermabrasion. I'm not too rigid: I won't do an area that actually has a pustule in it; however, if I have a patient who would otherwise be suitable but who keeps getting an occasional pimple here or there, that wouldn't stop me. To help prevent pimples that might interfere with the surgery, I might ask her or him to take tetracycline for a time before the dermabrasion.'

While acne is associated with adolescence, it can persist, with its attendant scars, even into middle age. Surgeons are less likely to recommend dermabrasion for patients forty years old or more who have acne scars. As we age, the skin becomes thinner, so the surgeon is more likely to suggest a face lift. One says, 'Even if the face lift dosen't help the acne scars, the fact that the skin is a little smoother from being pulled makes them a little less conspicuous.'

Hospitalisation

Many surgeons do dermabrasion on an outpatient basis; others prefer that their patients stay in hospital overnight.

Duration of Treatment

Usually, dermabrasion is done as a series of treatments over several months. Often there will be a total of three sessions for dermabrasion: first, the test; next, if the results are positive, the dermabrading of the scarred area of the face; after six months or a year, another session to dermabrade again in the same area in order to provide further improvement in the skin.

Anaesthesia

Dermabrasion is usually done under local anaesthetic in the United States of America, but most surgeons in the United Kingdom prefer to use a general anaesthetic.

Those who use local anaesthetic often give preoperative medication such as intravenous Valium.

Procedure

Surgeons use a motor-driven machine to power either a rapidly moving wire brush or a stone abrader.

If general anaesthetic isn't being used, a local anaesthetic will be injected into the face, or the face will be sprayed with a chemical that freezes it. Since the chemical action lasts only seconds, the face must be frozen and abraded in very small patches.

The surgeon goes over the skin with the abrader in as many directions as necessary.

Both during and after the procedure, which takes an hour or less, there will probably be a good deal of bleeding.

Aftermath

If you're not staying in hospital overnight, you'll be asked to have someone come along who can take you home. If the operation was done under local anaesthetic, you may be given a cup of tea or coffee and allowed to leave. If you had intravenous Valium, you'll probably be kept an hour—longer, if you still seem woozy.

There will be bandages over the area that's been dermabraded; the more extensive the area, the more bandages. The surgeon usually applies antibiotic ointment, medicated gauze, and then some outer gauze to catch the blood.

There will be swelling, sometimes severe. Some patients have such severe swelling around the mouth that they have to go on a liquid diet for two or three days.

Despite the blood, there isn't much pain associated with dermabrasion. The surgeon will probably recommend codeine or another non-aspirin painkiller for the first night.

Convalescence

You'll be out of work or school for a week to ten days after dermabrasion, primarily because you'll look terrible and wouldn't want the world to see you.

Some surgeons remove the bandages from your face after a day and have you use creams and/or soak your face in warm water after five days to soften the crust that forms; it usually then takes a few more days for the crust to fall off.

Other surgeons advise that the bandage be allowed to peel off, just like a scab, without any aid from either them or you. One surgeon tells his patients, 'If, within four or five days, it falls off by itself or is getting very loose so you can gently peel it off, you don't have to come to see me.' However, if it takes more than four or five days, the surgeon wonders whether he went too deep in dermabrading and usually prefers to remove the bandages personally.

When the bandages come off, your face will still be swollen and will look smoother than it will when it finally settles down after about a month. At the outset, the skin will be pink. It will probably be weeks or months before the 'permanent' colour manifests itself.

As soon as the bandages are off, cosmetics can be used, provided the skin has healed smoothly.

An important part of caring for dermabraded skin is to keep it out of the sun for six months. Whenever there is a chance of exposure to sun, be sure to wear a sun block and a brimmed hat. Many surgeons suggest having dermabrasion performed in the autumn or winter to minimise the chance of damage by sun rays.

Complications

There are four possible complications from dermabrasion. The most common is the formation of tiny whiteheads on the skin about a month after the procedure. They often disappear spontaneously; if not, the surgeon can easily eliminate them with an instrument designed for the purpose.

107

Very rarely, an area that has been dermabraded may appear infected (a genuine infection hardly ever occurs because of the good blood supply to the face) and require treatment with an antibiotic ointment.

As mentioned under 'Consultation', there is the possibility of permanent pigment change, which women can usually disguise with make up.

Finally, as with many of the surgical procedures we've discussed, there is the risk of developing raised scars. One of the reasons that many surgeons test an area of the skin before dermabrading is to learn whether raised scars will form.

Durability of Results

The results of dermabrasion are permanent. In the case of acne, another outbreak could, of course, lead to further scars.

As surgeons readily acknowledge, dermabrasion has its limitations. But it has proven effective in dealing with one of the problems of adolescence—acne scars—and some of the fine wrinkles that can be one of the unfortunate effects of ageing.

14 Other Skin Surgery

... colours that never fade ...
—Carrie Jacobs Bond

Besides the scarred or worn-looking skin that dermabrasion resurfaces and the fine lines that chemical skin
peeling erases or lessens, there are other skin conditions
that trouble people—and other techniques of cosmetic
surgery to combat them.

Birthmarks

Birthmarks are usually port-wine coloured and are
most commonly found on the head and neck. Most of the
traditional techniques, including medical tattooing (tattooing with a skin coloured pigment) and skin grafts,
have proved unsatisfactory. In some cases, the birthmark
can be cut out surgically in a series of operations in which
a bit is taken each time. There is some hope for a new
method—a series of treatments by laser— now beginning
to be used in the United States and the United Kingdom.
Cosmeticians report great success with cosmetics especially designed to cover port-wine birthmarks; these
cosmetics can be used even by young children.

109

Freckles

Facial freckles can be removed by dermabrasion. Freckles on the body can often be removed with an electric current.

Tattoos

The young man who has the name of a beloved tattooed on his chest or arm may live to regret the day—especially if he wants to get rid of that evidence of an old romance. The pigment used for a tattoo penetrates many layers of the skin. To remove a tattoo surgically, a series of operations may be required (as with a birthmark). To remove a large tattoo, a skin graft may be needed.

Xanthomas

Xanthomas are little deposits of fatlike material; they are usually yellowish and appear on the eyelids. They can be cut out or destroyed with an electric current. It is common for them to develop again.

15 Hair Transplants

If I live to be old, for I find I go down,
Let this be my fate in a country town;
May I have a warm house with a stone at the gate,
And a cleanly young woman to rub my bald pate.
— Walter Pope

William Higgins is a thirty-year-old salesman. He and his wife live in Brighton. On his second try at a hair transplant, he had successful results.

'I'd been losing my hair over about three or four years. What got to me most was that people were constantly stating the obvious: "You're losing your hair" or "You're going bald." It was beginning to rule my life. I had stopped socialising because of it.

'Very few people have a photograph of me from that time, because when I started losing my hair I wouldn't go anywhere near a camera—ever. When people got cameras out at a party or family gathering, I would just disappear, because I couldn't stand seeing what I looked like.

'I wouldn't say that looking younger was part of my motivation—though people now tell me I look ten years younger. It was just getting up in the morning, looking in the mirror, and not liking what I saw.

'I didn't consider a hairpiece. I have a cousin who wears one, and his looks terrible. Obviously, there are better wigs and poorer wigs, but seeing his just put me off. Even though a transplant costs more money, I decided to have it done.

'I went to my GP. He didn't know a doctor who did transplants, and he said, "Just face it; grin and bear it." I told him I was definitely going to do something about it, but he just said, "I'm not recommending you to anybody."

111

'Well, I got drunk one afternoon, and I thought, "I'm going to do something about it *now*." I had the "Dutch courage" to ring up a firm whose advertisements I'd seen in the paper and on the tube.

'I was living in Manchester then, so I went to a clinic there. But it didn't work out well at all. Because money was a big consideration, I had only a small amount done on the crown, and it didn't take very well. They say to leave it three months before you see any results, but after six months there still wasn't anything growing.

'When I went back to the clinic, they said, "Oh, we didn't guarantee it." They *had* said orally, "It's fully guaranteed," but I never got anything in writing. I've since learned that they weren't using qualified medical staff. Foolishly, I'd just gone to the first place I'd heard about.

'I still believed that hair transplanting would work if it was done properly, so when we moved to the south of England, I started looking for a clinic in London, as my work takes me there frequently. I visited five clinics to see if they would give me a guarantee. Only two would. Both offered a guarantee in writing that every graft they transplanted would produce a full amount of hair and that if it didn't, they would replace it. In fact, I've had two or three replaced.

'I asked about flap grafting because I'd heard of it, but I was put off mainly because of the cost. The clinic I chose said that there was no guarantee on flap grafting and that there is a high failure rate, so they don't recommend it. If a little graft fails, it can be replaced, but if a whole flap fails, you're left with a horrible inch-wide scar all around.

'So far I've had two punch-graft treatments with three months between. Each time I was in for about four hours. I wouldn't say it hurts; it was uncomfortable. The only thing I can compare it with is going to the dentist, and it's not as bad as that.

'They gave me some tablets about half an hour before they were going to start working, and then they froze the area with local anaesthetic. I didn't feel anything. Because the area is numb, all you can really feel is pressure. During the treatment, they told me all the time what they were doing: "Now we're taking the grafts out," etc.

"They kept me there for about an hour afterwards before they would let me drive home. They did a few tests to see what my reactions were and let me go when I was okay.

'I had a bandage on top and a little woolly sailor's hat that I wore over it, so no one could actually see. The bandage was on for two days, and then I returned to the clinic and they took it off.

'I went into our little pub with my woolly hat on. I've never worn a hat in my life before, but nobody said anything. Later, two or three people asked what I had had done, and I said, "I've had a small operation on my head," and that was that. Now that the hairs have grown through, I really don't mind telling people.

'While you've got the dressing on in the first few days, it isn't very pleasant sleeping, because it does feel a little tender. I remember once getting out of the car and banging my head—it hurt like hell.

'There were no big problems. They said that I shouldn't do any heavy exercise for about a week afterwards, that I shouldn't get my heart racing. And I had to be a little careful when I washed my hair. They gave me a special medicated shampoo, and I had to be careful to massage my hair gently and not get my nails in it.

'The little scabs lasted about two weeks, and they were the worst part. But I'd just pull my little hat on when I went to the pub. When the growth started, after two months, I got about half-an-inch a month.

'I wouldn't recommend anyone to go and have it done just because they're losing their hair. I know a lot of people who don't seem to mind. My father was almost identical to me, and he says he never thought about it at all.

'Anyone who does decide to have it done should check out the qualifications of the staff if they're having it done at a clinic. The current state of English law allows anyone to do an operation on anyone else, and unqualified people are taking advantage of this. I'd also be very sure to have a guarantee of results *in writing*.

113

'If I was back working at an office job instead of the freelance situation I have now, I'd have it done during my holidays. Otherwise everybody you saw would make remarks about your having it done. If you're particularly sensitive about it anyway, it's going to be that much worse for you. If you have it done before going on holiday, the scabs will all be gone when you get back.

'From the very beginning, I consulted with my wife. She thought I was mad, basically. I didn't have any reservations about the amount of money that had to be spent, but she did. Now she says there is a difference in me; I'm a more relaxed person and willing to go out again.

'We had to give up a lot to pay for the transplants. We sacrificed holidays. Normally I would change the car every two years, but we had to keep ours for longer than that. Our next car is going to be a soft-top—before, I didn't like going around with my head showing out of an open car, but now I can again.

'Altogether it cost nearly £1,300. I think it was well spent. In fact, knowing what I know now, I'd spend twice that much to have the same thing done.'

The story of William Higgins has a happy conclusion. But Michael Berry's attempts to renew his hair have spelled disaster. Berry lives in Leeds, is thirty-two and single, and drives a lorry for one of the nationally known breweries.

'Someone said that second to becoming impotent, a man fears the loss of his hair. This was certainly the case with me, and I can only say I regret my rash solution to the problem.

'I waited about six months after I noted significant hair loss, and then I began filling in adverts from the newspapers. I received confident replies that everything was possible and successful. In practice, this isn't the case, as I found out later. I finally chose a clinic with an international reputation—according to their advertisement. Since it's a large company, I presumed they must have had some success with the service they provided.

'I had an interview with a gentleman who prescribed a

114

number of grafts from the back of the head to be transplanted to the upper temple region. I paid an initial £35 as a guarantee that I would have the operation, and then, just before the transplant, I paid for sixty grafts at £5 per graft.

'The operation was carried out by a nurse. I had no prior knowledge of this, and I had naturally assumed that a doctor would do the operation. If I had known about that, I would have gone somewhere else. There was little pain during the operation, but it was very painful afterwards for several days.

'I was informed before and after the operation that any work on my hairline would be done free. When I returned to see them after six months, they were going to charge me. They said they just didn't believe that anyone at the clinic would have suggested in the first place that it would be a free part of the service.

'I can only say that the results of the transplant were very disappointing. I have a large cyst where the grafts were removed. When I showed the people at the clinic, they made no attempt to explain it, nor did they offer to do anything about it. They just said there was nothing to worry about.

'The grafts have been a constant embarrassment to me, as they show up so easily. There is very poor coverage on the part of my scalp where the transplant was done, so it's easily seen unless I cover it with my own hair. On a breezy day, that's very hard to do.

'I've seen several doctors who have expressed their disapproval of the quality of the transplant. I've even investigated having the transplant removed. One West End doctor told me he could do it without leaving a scar, but I've since learned that he was lying and that I would have scars if I had the transplant taken out.

'At the moment, I don't know what to do.'

Most men who begin to lose their hair feel a measure of Michael Berry's distress, especially those who begin to bald at an early age. It's little consolation to know that one in five men in the Western world loses hair.

115

Baldness is caused by a combination of heredity and hormones, and men tend to go bald in a predictable pattern: hair on the temples and crown may go, but it remains in the semi-circle around the back and sides from ear to ear (only very rarely do men lose hair there).

For a long time there was little remedy for baldness other than a hairpiece, with its attendant problems and possible embarrassment. About twenty-five years ago, an American doctor began transplanting hair-bearing follicles from the back and sides of the head, where the longest-lasting hair is found, to the temple and crown areas. Generally the body finds such transplants acceptable for blood, skin, and nerve supply, because the donor and recipient are the same person. Because the hair is taken from an area where the hair usually lasts for a lifetime, the results are relatively permanent; hair transplanted from there to the top will last as long as the hair on the sides and back remains. This method, called punch grafting, usually produces hair within about three months after the transplant, and the hair then grows at the normal rate of about one centimetre a month.

Opinion is divided as to the success rate of punch grafts. Many GPs and plastic surgeons estimate the success rate at fifty per cent. Spokesmen for major hair transplant clinics claim they are one hundred per cent successful.

Plastic surgeons admit that they don't like to do hair transplants because they find the procedure boring and time consuming.

More recently, another and more direct method of replacing lost hair has been developed. It's called the 'flap graft' and involves taking a hair-bearing flap (about three inches by six inches) from the side of the head above the ear and rotating it—with one end still attached to its original blood supply—across the bald area of the scalp. Up to three flaps can be rotated. The area in front of the flaps, where there will be a scar from the surgery, can be filled in with punch grafts.

The operation, done under general anaesthetic, takes between two hours and four and a half hours and requires hospitalisation for one to five nights. After leaving the hospital, patients spend one week to ten days at home before returning to work.

The advantage of this method, of course, is that you have hair immediately. The disadvantage, beside the fact that the cost is much higher than it is for punch grafting, is that it is very major surgery and has all the risks thereof. In fact the risks are compounded, because there is a major artery up the side of the neck in the area where the surgery takes place.

A London surgeon tells of a flap graft operation performed in the late 1970s by a Harley Street plastic surgeon. The patient was a thirty-year-old millionaire from North America. During the operation, he suffered cardiac arrest, apparently as the result of the faulty administration of the general anaesthetic. The surgeon finished the operation and then sent the patient off to a large London hospital, where they tried to revive him; but he had been reduced to the state of a vegetable. He was flown back to his home country, where he eventually died.

In discussing punch graft transplants, we're assuming that the patient is a Caucasian male who is having his own hair transplanted. Some clinics will treat women who have lost hair through scar tissue as the result of an accident; but in women, hair tends to thin all over, which means that there may be no good source of supply for transplanting. Surgeons say that it is also difficult to work on the hair of black patients. There is a problem in covering the donor site, because very curly hair is less manoeuvrable: it tends to grow straight out. Also, dark-skinned people are more prone to keloids—overgrowth of scar tissue that results in a lumpy-looking scar.

Generally, surgeons agree that artificial-hair implants, such as fibre implants and weaves are 'disasters', in terms of not only appearance, but also infections and other side effects. Journalist Lawrence Galton reported on twenty patients with fibre implants who were treated at the Cleveland, Ohio, Clinic Foundation: 'The victims had paid an average of $2,427 for their implants. Ten had developed infections; seventeen suffered from severe itching that didn't stop until the fibre fell out; eleven had scarring of the scalp. Nine had additional, permanent hair loss.'

In discussing hair transplants, we will be considering the widely accepted punch graft method.

Consultation

Whether you're seeing a plastic surgeon or using a hair transplant clinic, the consultant will want to know your medical background and will want to be sure that your expectations are realistic.

One of the major causes of complaint about hair transplants is that the patient expected to regain a full head of hair. Hair transplanting can't create new hair; it can only redistribute what you already have. With the finished product you will probably look as though your hair is thinning. The director of one clinic says, 'If patients accept that, fine. If they say, "I want it the way it was when I was eighteen," we could never satisfy them, no matter how many grafts we put in.' He goes on to comment on hairpiece wearers: 'If a person is a hair piece wearer and he thinks the transplant is going to look anything like that hairpiece, there's no way we will treat him. His own hair didn't look like the hairpiece originally.'

After being sure your expectations are realistic, the next issue will be your general health—particularly the state of your heart and the names of any drugs you may be taking for heart problems. The reason for this concern is that the local anaesthetic used for the transplant has vaso-constrictors, which make the blood coagulate, and heart patients may be taking anticoagulants.

Next to your general health, the most important concern is your donor hair, the hair available on the back and sides of the head to be used for the donor grafts. Both quantity and quality of hair are important. The surgeon will want a minimum of six to ten hairs in a four-millimetre graft. With less than that there's reduced density and the coverage won't be as good. Dark, coarse hair is ideal—much better than blond, fine hair. Blond hair is often so close to the colour of the scalp that coverage isn't good, but dark, coarse hair gives both good appearance and good coverage.

A clinic may require that you take a physical examination there, whereas a hospital-affiliated plastic surgeon may require only a recommendation from your GP. In either case, the doctor will want to know about heart conditions, tendency to bleed, allergy to any drugs, and blood or scalp disorders (which would have to be cleared up before a transplant).

As a prospective patient, you will want some important information. First, does the clinic or surgeon guarantee the results of the transplant? (If not, consider looking elsewhere for someone who does.) Second, who will be doing the surgery? Be *absolutely sure* that the work is being done by a surgeon.

Hair transplants can only rarely be done on NHS.

Preferred Age

The patient must be old enough so that the baldness pattern is clearly established. Most people who seek hair transplants are between twenty-eight and forty.

A clinic consultant says, 'We really don't like doing grafts before an applicant is twenty or twenty-one, and even then you've got to be very careful. A patient may be receding only at the temple area, and you can't really estimate the total amount of his baldness in the future.

'So we've got to examine his hair and treat him only if his hair in the rear section is very, very good, with no sign of thinning at all. If we've any doubts, we tell him to come back later. Here's the problem: obviously we can expect him to recede slightly more; that's okay for a small area, because he will have ample donor sites. But if he recedes the whole way—very low on the crown—he wouldn't have enough donor site to fill in.

'The patient has to understand that if he starts having treatment around the temples and he recedes and loses more hair, he's obligated himself to further treatment, because it would look silly to have transplanted hair, a

119

gap, and then his own, naturally grown, hair. The critical factor with young people is trying to ascertain how much hair they will lose.'

Some clinics and hospital-connected surgeons will not accept patients over sixty because of the additional risks attendant upon their age.

Hospitalisation

Transplants by the punch-graft method are done on an outpatient basis. Each treatment will probably involve your spending four to five hours at the clinic or surgery, because you won't be able to leave until the blood has congealed and the anaesthetic worn off. During the wait after the surgery, you can have a cup of tea, read, watch television.

Whatever the size of the area, you'll need at least two treatments. Someone with complete baldness of the temple and crown would probably need four treatments. There is a minimum of one month between treatments, but you can space them as far apart as you like.

Anaesthesia

The treatments are done under local anaesthetic. Usually you will be given a sedative about half an hour before the treatment begins. Some patients find that they don't need a sedative after the first treatment because they aren't apprehensive anymore.

Local anaesthetic will be used in two areas: the donor site, from which the grafts are taken, and the recipient site, into which they are planted.

Procedure

The usual procedure is to make a parting across the back of the head in the donor site. The surgeon then removes pieces of skin with hair roots attached. The grafts may be removed in a row and the skin at the donor site stitched

120

together; or they may be spaced at noncontiguous intervals and the skin left to heal naturally. In either case, your hair can be combed over the donor site immediately so that stitches or scarring won't be visible.

After removing the grafts from the donor site, the surgeon will take matching circles of between two and five millimetres from the recipient site and put a graft—'plug' —into each. 'It's like putting a cork in a bottle,' says one surgeon.

The plugs have to be spaced so they are not touching, because each needs its own blood supply. (This is why two treatments are required, even for a small site.)

The number of grafts transplanted at a single treatment depends on the area being treated. The average is fifty to one hundred grafts.

Aftermath

After the treatment you'll have a turbanlike bandage on your head, covering both the donor and recipient areas. You'll usually be given a sailor-style cap to cover the bandage, which will remain in place for twenty-four to forty-eight hours. If necessary, you can then remove it yourself, but most surgeons and clinics prefer to have it removed by professionals, if it's possible for you to return to their surgery or clinic.

Convalescence

The hardest part of having a punch-graft transplant is enduring the three weeks when you have crusts on your head—and then waiting for your transplanted hair to surface. It's approximately three months after the operation that hair starts to grow through, so you have all that time to look into the mirror and wonder what's happening. Then hair should begin to grow naturally at the rate of your own hair, usually about one centimetre a month.

You'll probably be told that you can wash your hair for the first time five days after the treatment—as long as you

121

keep hands off the recipient site. You may be given a specially medicated shampoo or told to buy a mild baby shampoo. Ten days following surgery, you'll be able to wash your whole head.

Scars

For about three weeks there will be small crusts formed over each graft. When the crusts come off, the skin tone is slightly pinkish and gradually fades to match the surrounding skin. If before the procedure you had some hair on the crown or at the temples, you can change your hairstyle to cover the crusts. If you have been wearing a hairpiece, you can continue to wear your wig so the spots won't be seen. But if you were bald, you can't cover up and will have to accept visible scarring after each treatment for the two or three weeks it lasts.

One clinic consultant says, 'The easiest thing is to be honest about it and let people know you've had a transplant. If you don't want to tell anyone, the best solution is to have the transplant when you're going on holiday. Especially if you go on holiday in the sun, there's nothing odd about wearing a sun hat. Besides, you know that the people you'll meet probably are people you'll never see again.'

Complications

Apart from the inconvenience of the convalescence, there shouldn't be any complications. The biggest problem with hair transplants comes from grafts that don't 'take'. A reputable surgeon or clinic will replace them without charge.

Durability of Result

The transplanted hair will last as long as the hair at the

donor site lasts—and, as noted earlier, the hair on the sides and back of the head is the last to go.

Not many men are easily philosophical about the loss of their hair. It is often their 'crowning glory', an important element in their self-image, and the loss of it is a psychologically difficult experience.

Men who don't want to go through the discomfort or expense of a hair transplant might look to Telly Savalas and Yul Brynner as examples. Both men's stardom probably has something to do with the strong sexuality they project. So a man might consider flaunting his baldness, and take it *all* off.

16 Electrolysis

You should be women, and yet your beards forbid me to interpret That you are so.—William Shakespeare

Adolescence, a time of physical and emotional turbulence, becomes downright miserable when we're the target of teasing by others. When Margaret Chase, now twenty-two and a receptionist at a television station, developed facial hair growth as an adolescent, she turned to electrolysis for help.

'When I was thirteen, I started growing a mustache. It was quite bad, and it was black. Boys would tease me about it. I didn't like to sit in bright lights—especially as my face was spotty as well.

'I went to a local clinic, but I was told that I had to be menstruating regularly for a year before they'd do electrolysis.

'I used to wax and cream my mustache, which created a problem when I came back at sixteen for treatment. They still weren't too keen to work on me, but they started off gradually to see how it responded, and it was all right. Where I had waxed or creamed there was a tendency for the hair to regrow even after electrolysis.

'When I decided to have it done, I was scared, but I thought it would be worth it. The treatment hurt more than I imagined. It is painful, and it made me sneeze while it was being done. The treatments for the lip lasted about twenty minutes at first; towards the end, they were just ten minutes.

'For about two weeks after, there were painful little

lumps on the skin and a few tiny spots with pus in them. I had been ordered not to squeeze them, but I did anyway.

'The treatment took several months, but was very successful, and I can't tell you what a relief it was to get rid of that hair. Now I'm back to have the bikini-line hair removed. These treatments last about half an hour, because that's all the suffering I can stand. Where the hair's been removed, there are little blisters. There's a sting when they put the needle in for the bikini-line treatments, because they turn the needle up more.

'Even though it hurts, it's really well worth it to have the hair gone. I'm going to have my legs done next.'

Margaret Chase was embarrassed by her hair growth, but Thelma Duffy, a twenty-four-year-old factory worker from London's East End, came to a clinic mainly because she was sick of the inconvenience of shaving her legs regularly and wanted to be rid of the hair growth once and for all.

'I'm having the treatment out of vanity. I got fed up with shaving, but I think it's unfeminine to have bristly legs. I used to shave my legs on a Friday night, and then I'd have to shave them again on Sunday—and I really hated it.

'I used creams, but they're messy and they smell. I wanted a permanent way to get rid of the hair, and I thought a couple of years of discomfort would be worth it.

'Most of my friends shave their legs, and they think I'm very brave to have this done. I haven't told my mother, because she wouldn't approve of this way of spending my money.

'When I came for the consultation, they checked my skin and hair type; I have very strong, dark hair. Then they gave me the option of a half-hour treatment.

'I've been having the treatment for a year now, and it will take another year. At this stage I come in for four treatments every six weeks. For the first six months I really thought it was a waste of time, because they can only do a small patch at a time.

'There's discomfort, but it doesn't hurt. For ten days to

125

two weeks, blood spots come up and stay for two weeks. They look like pinpricks. For the first twenty-four hours after treatment, I have to put on a lotion every four hours. I get a sort of burning sensation, because I have naturally sensitive skin.

'I wear trousers to cover the blood spots. But I'm a bit worried with summer coming—I can't wear trousers all the time. If I go out in a skirt, I wear dark stockings.

'It's also a problem going out with a boyfriend; I can't really spend the night. One boyfriend thought I was mad. A second didn't take much notice but stayed clear of my legs. For four months now, I've been seeing someone else pretty seriously; he has seen my legs, and he says, "If that's what you want, do it."

'I didn't have second thoughts about the money. I earn good money doing shift work, and it's something I'm doing because I want to.'

One of the ironies in the relationship of the sexes is that men often lose hair they'd like to keep, and women often acquire hair they'd prefer not to have.

There are many causes of such hair growth: heredity; hormones (endocrine disorder); race (for example, Italian, Spanish, and Persian women often have low hairlines); drugs taken for other medical conditions; stress; and birth control pills.

Unwanted hair growth is also associated with three times in women's lives that involve substantial hormonal changes: puberty, pregnancy, and menopause.

The hair growth that women most often seek to have removed is on the face, usually over the upper lip. Other common sites of unwanted hair are the breast, around the nipples; and the bikini line (at the inner thighs in the pubic area). Growth in both places is often encouraged by the use of birth control pills.

Some types of unwanted hair are embarrassing. Others, such as underarm and leg hair, are less embarrassing than inconvenient; many Western women are accustomed to removing hair in these areas for aesthetic reasons.

Whatever your reasons for wanting to be rid of hair,

there is a permanent method of removing it—electrolysis. Most NHS hospitals have electrolygists on their staff; but their work is usually limited to those who have severe (usually hormonal) problems, and a referral from a dermatologist is usually required. In most major cities, however, there are clinics that specialise in electrolysis.

Consultation

One of the first things you'll want to know is just what electrolysis can and can't do—and what persons are poor risks.

A consultant explains: 'We can do the upper lip, the bikini line, breast hair, low hairlines, and hair on the nape of the neck. We can also do leg hair, but it can be painful because of the padding of flesh.

'We can't do hair in the nose or ears, because these are sensitive areas that can become infected. We don't do hair under the eyebrows, because it's too risky—imagine what could happen if someone moves. We don't do pubic hair or hair on darker-pigmented areas, because there the hair is deep-rooted and so the procedure is painful. Nor do we treat hair *on* the lips or *on* the nipples or in the genital areas, because those are very sensitive areas.'

There is some controversy about whether to do electrolysis on underarm hair. Some clinics will do it; others won't, because the primary sweat glands are located in the underarm and could be damaged by the electric needle.

There are also medical conditions that make clinics either discourage treatment or refuse it outright. Those with heart conditions or diabetes would be treated only with a letter from their GP that it's not a medical risk; those with severe acne, eczema, or psoriasis need to have those conditions cleared up before treatment can begin; and no one with hepatitis can be treated.

The consultant will want to know your medical background and the cause of the problem. If a medical condition is causing the excess hair, you may be referred to a GP or an endocrinologist. The consultant will also want to know if you're taking any hormones, because such therapy should be completed before electrolysis is started.

Another important consideration is what you may have done in the past to get rid of unwanted hair. One consultant discusses the problems caused by such efforts: 'Facial hair becomes different if clients pluck, wax, cream, or shave it. Plucking destroys the roots but can create secondary roots. Waxing is similar; it's mass plucking, and it takes out the fine down—hair that doesn't need to be taken out. If you remove the fine down, you take away the skin's protection, leaving it dry and bare-looking. And waxing can encourage the growth of a beard, just as regular plucking does.

'Depilatory cream is a version of the chemical used to perm hair. It's a permanent carried to excess in that it breaks off the hair completely. It can do damage to the skin and make it more sensitive. As to shaving: men shave and their beards get stronger. But it's the least-bad thing to do.

'If you use tweezers or wax, you strengthen the hair. It's the most natural thing for the body to repair itself.'

Consultations at most clinics are free. Some consultants will offer to remove one hair at no cost, to convince you that the pain is minimal. Often, at the end of the consultation, you'll be offered the option of a half-hour treatment, usually at full cost.

Electrolygists require their clients to pledge that they will do nothing to the hair on their own while undergoing treatment.

In some cases (for example, when the problem is hormonal), electrolysis can be done on NHS.

Preferred Age

Most electrolygists won't treat anyone under sixteen, and, like those at the clinic Margaret Chase visited, they want the client to have menstruated regularly for one full year, indicating that any hormonal changes have been resolved.

Hospitalisation

Electrolysis is done on an outpatient basis.

Duration of Treatments

Time required to remove the hair varies with the individual. One consultant said, 'Treatments usually start with a session of half an hour every fortnight. Later we go to ten minutes every six weeks—even to ten minutes every three months. Treatments on the sensitive upper lip are only about fifteen minutes long. After each treatment the hair gets weaker and finer, but you can't predict the rate of change.

'The hair growth cycle is different on different parts of the body, and we have to wait for the hair to grow through before we can treat it again. For example, the hair growth cycle (roots to surface) on the legs is two months, so, at most, we can treat each hair six times in one year. That's one reason it takes up to two years to remove leg hair permanently.'

Anaesthesia

Electrolygists can give a local anaesthetic, but most don't like to, and some won't. The usual local anaesthetic for electrolysis is a spray. Part of its activity is to close the pores, which makes treatment more difficult, because the action of electrolysis is to take something from open pores.

Procedure

With a tiny electric needle, the electrolygist passes a fine current down the side of the hair into the follicle. The needle does not pierce the skin, because it goes into an open hole—the pore. In the process, heat is released that coagulates the capillaries. Nourishment to the hair is blocked, and that inhibits its growth. With each treatment, part of the food sac is killed, so the hair gets

129

weaker and weaker until it stops growing altogether.

According to electrolygists, there isn't any pain—though they admit that depends on the individual pain threshold. At most, they say, you'll feel the heat and, possibly, a sensation like a pinprick.

However, many people who have undergone treatment say they've experienced some pain or discomfort from electrolysis; but they add that the duration of the pain is very brief.

Aftermath

There is often a difference of opinion between clinic spokespersons and clients about aftereffects, as there is about pain. Clinic representatives say that there are no physical aftereffects, though the skin reacts very slightly, especially greasy skin and fair, fine skin.

Clients, however, often report the appearance of blisters and or blood spots that remain for a few weeks after each treatment. You will probably want to restrict the kind of clothing you wear as well as your activities: with blisters showing , you can't very well wear shorts or a bathing suit.

Convalescence

There is no period of convalescence, and no time lost from work as a result of electrolysis. (In fact some people come for treatment during their lunch hours.)

Scars

There are no scars, as such, after electrolysis. However, sometimes electrolysis enlarges pores noticeably, a factor that should be weighed in deciding whether to have such treatment. Some people might prefer to shave an upper lip rather than to risk looking 'pitty' there.

Durability of Results

Electrolysis destroys the unwanted hair permanently.

Men and Electrolysis

Far less often than women do, men also have hair removed by electrolysis. Some have treatment for hair at the back of the shoulders, or for permanent removal of their beards. Those who come for beard removal are usually between eighteen and thirty. Some are allergic to razors and must either remove their beards completely or grow a full beard. Others just don't want to shave.

Clinics are often reluctant to treat men, partly because women clients are embarrassed in the reception area when men are also there. Another problem is that, because the male beard is so deeply rooted, the duration of treatment is extensive and is more painful than is most of the work done on women.

Electrolysis resembles hair transplanting in that both are series of treatments occurring over a period of time. Growing hair and killing hair are both long processes requiring experts to do the work and clients who have the patience to await appreciable results.

131

17 Protruding Ears Correction

I believe they talked of me, for they laughed consumedly.
—George Farquhar

Irene Shaw is twenty-three and a flight attendant for a major airline. She is the oldest of four children and lives with her father and three brothers in Hounslow.

'I was born with "bat ears" like my mother, and my youngest brother, Matthew, has the same problem. My other two brothers have ears flat against their head, just like my father.

When I was small, I always wanted to wear my hair pulled back, but my mother would say, "No, it doesn't suit you," and brush it over my ears. When I was seven or eight, I would stop before I reached school and tie my hair back. Once, when we were out in the school yard, one of the boys said, "What time does the next flight take off?" and made flapping motions with his hands behind his ears. I was crushed. For the first time I realized why my mother had kept my hair hiding my ears.

'There was no question of my having surgery on my ears; there simply wasn't the money. But I decided I would earn it some day.

'Then my brother Matthew was born, and he had the same problem; the two boys born in between had normal ears.

'As soon as she knew about Matthew's problem, our mother decided to take a job so that there would be the money for him to have the surgery before he went to school. Unfortunately, she died two years ago. She had saved about half the money, but my father couldn't really see the need for the operation. He said, "Ears are for hearing, and Matthew can hear." But he no longer objected when I said that I would pay for the half that mother's savings didn't cover. I couldn't bear to have Matthew experience what I had that time in the school yard, and I thought I could wait another year or two to have my ears done.

'When Matthew was just five, I took him to our GP, who agreed that there was a problem; we then went for a consultation with a plastic surgeon. The surgeon was careful to be sure that Matthew wanted to have the surgery done. He asked Matthew if anything about his appearance bothered him, and Matthew said, "Do you mean my ears? I know they stick out and look funny."

'Matthew was scheduled for surgery; he stayed in hospital overnight. He had a general anaesthetic, because he's an active child and the surgeon felt the operation would be more successful that way.

'We had two problems after Matthew came home. He was rather grumpy about sleeping with an elastic band around his head, and he developed a slight infection, which was cleared up quickly with antibiotics. And he didn't understand why he couldn't play football with the other boys at once.

'I would say that Matthew's operation was a success, and when he starts school soon, he'll be spared the teasing I had.'

The same child who will part with a favourite toy to ease a friend's unhappiness might heedlessly injure a playmate with protruding ears by calling her or him 'Dumbo' or 'Donkey Ears'.

When parents hear their children's tearful reports of such taunts, or when they chance to overhear the hurtful name-calling, often they seek out a plastic surgeon to correct the problem ears. Adults whose protruding ears were not corrected in childhood also seek out this surgery.

Correction of protruding ears, commonly called bat

ears, can often be done when a child is only four or five years old, because by that time the ear has reached ninety per cent of its adult growth. If the operation is done too early, there could be damage to the covering of the ear cartilage.

A plastic surgeon says, 'Today bat ears are not such a problem as they were before the mid-1960s. With short hair, if the ears stuck out, everyone knew it. Now most people's ears are covered by their hair.

'There are two major types of protruding ears. The first is caused by the absence of the antihelix, the extra fold in the ear that gives the ear its shape. The second is caused by an over-large concha [the shell-shaped opening inside the ear]. When that's too big, it will make the ear stick out in the shape of a cup.

'I think more girls have the surgery done than boys, even though the boys' hair would be shorter. Girls are just more sensitive to that type of malformation; and when they become adolescents, they may want to wear their hair behind their ears.

'When the surgery is done on adults, the actual operation is the same. Adults may need more pain medicine than children, because they tend to be more conscious of pain. On the other hand, children need a sturdier dressing, and they probably require more reassurance.'

Consultation

If the candidate for the procedure is under ten or eleven, the surgeon will probably see the child in the company of one or both parents. A plastic surgeon explains, 'Young children are uncomfortable without their parents; and the interaction of parents and child is revealing to the surgeon. Most parents who are forcing a child to have an operation are so oblivious of having that motivation that they wouldn't even think I'd be looking for it. But there's enough honesty and naivete on the part of the child to give me an accurate assessment of the situation.

'To justify surgery, it's not enough that the child *has* bat ears. The child must be *bothered* by them; the parents must be sensitive and understanding. By the time they're seven or eight, children have a concept of appearance, both of face and body, so they can participate in the judgement. What the operation offers the child is freedom from ridicule.

'If a child is to have the surgery, it's often a good idea to schedule it for a school holiday period, preferably one other than summer. Usually children don't want their friends to see them with the dressing on, so they'll want to be at home after the surgery—but many are reluctant to miss summer activities, even for the short time necessary.'

A GP may recommend that the surgery be done on NHS for the psychological advantages it offers a child. The surgery is, however, purely cosmetic; bat ears do not present a hearing problem.

Preferred Age

Surgeons say that, from the physical point of view, the best age for the operation is about fourteen, when the ear has almost reached its maximum growth. However, they believe that the psychological benefits of having the surgery done before the child enters primary school are so significant that they recommend scheduling such surgery before a child is subject to teasing from classmates.

Hospitalisation

The usual hospital stay is one night. If the operation is done under local anaesthetic, often the patient may go home the day of the surgery.

Anaesthesia

Most plastic surgeons use general anaesthetic on young children, who may not cooperate reliably under local anaesthetic. With adolescents and adults, a surgeon

135

explains, 'I can usually tell when they're in for the consultation whether they are stable enough to cooperate with a local anaesthetic.

Procedure

The two major types of bat ears are corrected by slightly different procedures. In neither case is the hair touched, or the inner ear. In both cases the incision is made in the back of the ear. A plastic surgeon explains, 'Originally, only skin was removed from behind the ear, and the ear was pulled back, but in time the cartilage would spring back out, so the problem wouldn't be solved permanently. Plastic surgeons became aware that you really had to do something about the carilage. A Swedish plastic surgeon, Tord Skoog, found that if you injured the cartilage in a controlled fashion by scratching it, you could get a pleasingly rounded contour. This operation is the best way to deal with the absence of the antihelix.

'For the other problem, where the concha is too big and so causes a cup ear, basically all that's done is to remove a crescent-shaped piece of cartilage and also some skin.'

Either operation takes about one hour.

Aftermath

After the operation, the patient will be wearing a compression dressing that goes around the whole head and is either wrapped under the chin or wound like a turban. The dressing will stay on for five to ten days, though some surgeons prefer to put on a lighter dressing after a day or two.

There is often considerable swelling, but it disappears in a few weeks.

There is little pain after the operation, and the discomfort patients experience can be controlled by codeine.

Convalescence

The patient usually sees the surgeon after five days to have some of the stitches removed and to have a lighter dressing put on, if this wasn't done earlier. All the stitches are usually out after five to ten more days.

A plastic surgeon says, 'The reason for keeping the head wrap on children is so that they won't scratch their ears while sleeping, or injure them when running. For at least a month, there should be no swimming and diving activities that would create compression against the ears. But they can run and play. If parents and child use common sense, the child can pretty much go back to normal activity. Adults can resume normal activities after a day or two, though the strictures on swimming and diving apply to them also.'

For several weeks after the head wrap is removed, patients sleep with an elastic band—much like those that skiers wear—around the head.

In addition to the swelling, there may be discolouration and numbness that may last for several weeks.

After a week, patients can wash their hair.

The only other restriction is that the ears not be exposed to extreme heat or cold for six weeks after the surgery.

Scars

Since the incisions are made behind the ear in both operations, there are no visible scars.

Complications

A plastic surgeon explains, 'In all plastic surgery, we want the patients to know potential problems beforehand. If the patient is a child, it's important that the parents understand what problems may arise, because children have no concept of complications.

'The three major complications are haematoma [a collection of blood under the skin], infection, and skin slough. For haematoma, the surgeon takes out a couple of

137

stitches and removes the blood collected under the skin. For infection, the patient is given antibiotics, and any pus that collects is drained out. For skin slough, which could be caused by the dressing being too tight, you just wait until it heals on its own.

'Actually, the complication that I've most often seen after this operation is that the result isn't very good. That is caused if the surgeon isn't skilful enough. When done by a competent, well-trained plastic surgeon, the results are very good in the majority of cases.'

Our playmates and growing friendships with them are one of the major joys of childhood. But playmates can be a source of pain for children who are 'different'—whether the difference be race, a speech problem, or a physical imperfection, however small. Children born with bat ears can become the butts of jokes; they are, however, more fortunate than most other children with physical problems, because the condition can be corrected easily through surgery.

18 Squints Correction

A weary time! a weary time!
How glazed each weary eye.
—Samuel Coleridge Taylor

Mildred Tuttle teaches in the fifth form in a Salisbury school; her husband, John, is also a teacher. Their daughter Nancy underwent surgery to correct a squint. Her mother describes the process.

'I first noticed Nancy's eye turning when she was just under three. I was dreadfully afraid that something might be wrong with her vision; I'm sure anyone would be concerned, but my husband and I are great readers and would have hated our daughter being unable to share our pleasure.

'I took Nancy to an ophthalmologist, and his diagnosis was "lazy eye". He said that he would treat it by putting a patch over her good eye for a time and then operating after the vision in the lazy eye had strengthened. He said that the operation might get the eyes to function as a unit and would certainly improve their appearance.

'During the time her good eye was patched, I felt like a policeman. She's a very active and curious child and kept wanting to remove the patch to look at her picture books or at the television.

'The treatment was successful, and by the time she was three and a half, the vision in her lazy eye had strengthened to the point that the surgeon scheduled the operation.

'Our hospital didn't have arrangements for a parent to stay overnight, but John and I stayed with Nancy until

139

after she was asleep the night before the surgery, and we were back very early in the morning. She was very good, though I'm sure she was more than a bit frightened. The surgeon told her that she wasn't to use her eyes for the first three days; that meant she couldn't look at any of her books or watch television. John and I told endless stories to keep her amused during those days.

'She recuperated very quickly, and was soon back to playing with her little friends. Unfortunately, her eyes were overcorrected; her eye now turns out. The surgeon has assured us that she can have a second operation fairly soon to take care of that problem. Even if she weren't to have the second operation, she looks much better than she did before.'

When Nancy was born, Mildred Tuttle's first concern, like many parents, was whether she was normal. Assured that her daughter had the right number of fingers and toes and all organs in the proper places, she breathed a sigh of relief. However, the eye condition that developed later could have set Nancy apart from other children and—like the bat ears discussed in the previous chapter—subjected her to the taunts of playmates and schoolfellows.

Squints can be either convergent (one or both eyes turned in) or divergent (one or both eyes turned out). Some cultures have regarded squints, especially the divergent squint, as very attractive. The ancient Greeks so valued the outward-turned gaze that they would cut the muscle on the inside of the eye with a flint in order to achieve it. Though the divergent squint can be beautiful, most people agree that a convergent squint can make one look very unpleasant.

An ophthalmologist explains that both difficulties are caused by problems in the binocular function—that is, the eyes working together as a unit. But he adds that seeing with just one eye isn't the problem many people think. 'Binocular single vision is a wildly overrated commodity. Except for an international tennis player, an airline pilot, a surgeon, or someone in a comparable occupation, most people can do without it nicely. It mustn't be confused with depth perception. You can perceive depth with one eye. You get better depth perception with two eyes, but you can function perfectly happily without stereoscopic vision. Of course, there may be good social reasons for surgical correction.'

There are two main factors causing convergent squints. Some children are born with a defect in binocular function, though nobody is quite sure why. Their eyes don't function as a pair, and usually one eye turns in. An ophthalmologist says, 'It is presumed that the child gets double vision, and the body doesn't like this. It therefore suppresses the image in the turning eye, and that eye then becomes what we call a lazy eye. A lazy eye is one that doesn't see, rather than one that doesn't move properly. With this condition, it's not that one eye is wrong and the other okay: it's the *pair* that's wrong.'

Lazy eye, the most common type of squint, usually comes on between age two and a half and age four, and it nearly always requires the wearing of a patch before surgery. The good eye is patched to make the lazy eye work, and once the lazy eye has sight, the eyes can be strengthened surgically. Surgeons know after a month whether the patch treatment is working. If it is, the child will have to continue to wear the patch until the surgery, because otherwise the vision in the lazy eye weakens again.

An ophthalmologist says, 'When you straighten the eyes surgically, you hope that they will function as a unit, but that wish is not granted as often as we'd like. Although you straighten the lazy eye, the eyes may not function perfectly as a pair. But the patient will not have double vision, and the result may be excellent cosmetically.'

The second type of childhood squint is called 'congenital alternators'. Children with this condition are born with squints and will never have binocular function, but they have good vision in each eye. If they fix upon an object with the left eye, the right eye will squint, and vice versa. Says an ophthalmologist, 'The operation for this condition is cosmetic, and there may be good personal or psychological reasons to do it. With lazy eye, we are trying to correct both function and appearance; with congenital

141

alternators, it is just appearance.'

Squints not corrected in childhood can be corrected in later years. Sometimes adults acquire squints—usually through lesions to the nerves; sometimes to the muscles. An ophthalmologist explains, 'Children with congenital alternators *don't have* double vision; those with lazy eye *suppress* double vision. But if an adult has a squint, he or she has double vision that can't be suppressed. The only way to eliminate that double vision without surgery would be to cover one eye. The causes in adults are usually accidents—automobile or tennis, for example—or a vascular problem like high blood pressure.'

Consultation

As soon as parents notice a persistent squint in their child, they should seek advice from an ophthalmologist, who will advise on the best course of treatment. Approximately half of all squints respond to nonsurgical treatment, such as the wearing of eyeglasses and the use of special eyedrops. In the other fifty percent of cases, the surgeon will recommend surgical correction for functional and/or cosmetic purposes.

The surgeon will have to assess how much deviation there is and whether one eye or both eyes should be operated on. In the case of lazy eye, only that one eye requires surgery.

The surgeon will want to study the child's eye muscles very carefully to decide on a proper course of action. He or she will judge which of the six eye muscles are too weak, which are normal, and which are overdoing their role.

Sometimes children who have very wide epicanthic folds (the folds alongside the nose) will be brought to an ophthalmologist for consultation. When a child with this wide fold of skin looks to the side, the eye nearest the nose looks as though it's turned in too far. But this child doesn't need treatment: when the nose grows, the epicanthic fold gets taken up and the eyes look—and are, as they have been—straight.

142

Preferred Age

You should discuss with the ophthalmologist the ideal time for treatment. Surgery can be done on the eyes of children as young as six months, and many surgeons believe that the earlier the surgery is done, the better the chance for improvement in function. An ophthalmologist says, 'We will guide the parents as to what we think the best time is. We try to do the surgery before children are of school age.

'If you take babies in under the age of two, they hardly know what's happening to them. With children of five or six, you can explain what's happening, and they're usually quite good. The children who are awkward are those between age two and a half and age four and a half. They're aware that they're away from home, and they know what's happening is unpleasant, but they can't comprehend the situation. For that reason many hospitals try to offer accommodation to mothers.

Hospitalisation

The child will usually be hospitalised for two or three nights. A few surgeons will operate for squints on an outpatient basis.

Anaesthesia

General anaesthesia is used on children. Adults can have the surgery under a local anaesthetic, but many elect general anaesthesia.

Procedure

The surgeon repositions muscles at both corners of the eye. The muscles are outside the eyeball, so it does not have to be incised. Thus there is almost no danger of loss of vision.

One muscle is loosened and the other tightened (depending on the nature of the squint), and each is

143

reattached to the eye in a position that allows the eye to turn in the direction necessary to align eyes. There will be two stiches in each muscle.

The operation takes about one hour.

The incisions are underneath the eyelid, so the scar is minimal.

Aftermath

The eye operated on will be red, swollen, and tender. The use of bandages varies from surgeon to surgeon. Some don't bandage the eyes at all; if only one eye was operated on, some put a pad on that eye for a day or two. Very few surgeons bandage both eyes anymore.

For the first few days, ophthalmologists usually apply eye ointments and cold compresses.

There may be discomfort after the operation, but it is usually tolerated easily with aspirin.

Convalescence

Surgeons and ophthalmologists agree that children bounce back very quickly from the surgery. For the first three or four days they are to rest their eyes and not read or watch television. For about two weeks they shouldn't engage in vigorous sports such as bicycling or swimming. For up to six months the eye operated on will continue to get very red after swimming. Apart from this special circumstance, the swelling and redness are usually gone after one or two weeks.

Complications

One 'complication' can be that the correction is imperfect. An ophthalmologist estimates that about thirty percent of patients are either undercorrected or overcorrected (so that they go from a convergent squint to a divergent one, or vice versa). A second operation can resolve this problem. The difficulty is usually due to muscle tone, a factor over which the operating physician or surgeon has no control.

Some surgeons deliberately undercorrect a convergent squint, since our eyes diverge very slightly as we grow.

One ophthalmologist says, 'You can do the same correction on three different children, and one might be perfect, one might be overcorrected, and one might be undercorrected. People are different, and they react differently.'

As with most surgery, there is the possibility of infection; usually that can be cleared up with antibiotic treatment in a week or two.

The patient may also get reddish fibrous tissue of about the thickness of mucous membrane about a quarter of an inch behind the cornea. Such tissue is usually easily excised.

The most serious complication, which is also extremely rare, is perforation of the eye when the surgeon inserts the needle into the eye wall to stitch the muscles. (The eye wall at the incision point is about .3 millimetre thick, about the thickness of your fingernail.) Should this perforation occur, the patient has either an intraocular haemorrhage or retinal detachment. In case of the first, the surgeon can apply a nitrogen-filled probe that creates a scar tissue reaction on the inside of the eye to seal the hole. If there's a retinal detachment, another operation will be done within about three weeks.

Durability of Result

Surgeons say that for about seventy percent of patients, one operation solves the problem permanently. In many cases the surgeon will have an idea of the probable duration of the operation's effects. An ophthalmologist says, 'I see a patient at least three or four times before the surgery. If the degree of variation from the preoperative condition is the same during all of those visits, the chances are very good for a long-term result. With patients who have a different degree of variance on each visit, it's difficult to predict the durability of the adjustment. In some cases it may last just a few years; in others, ten to twenty years.'

145

As to the success rate of surgery for squints, an ophthalmologist says, 'You have to consider whether "success" is a matter of functional result or appearance result. If you're talking about functional result, then the operation's success rate is probably low—much lower than we would like to admit. We operate on a lot of squints thinking that we are correcting the function, but the eyes do not work together as a pair, so it turns out to be a cosmetic operation. The *cosmetic* operation to straighten the eyes is almost always successful.'

When children are very young, their sense of self-image comes from their parents, who wouldn't hurt a child by calling attention to a physical imperfection. However, as children grow older, more of their self-image is derived from their peers, and the frankness of other children can inflict terrible pain on a child whose appearance has even a minor blemish. Fortunately for the child whose problem is a squint, the appearance problem can be remedied—usually before the child has had to bear the brunt of others' jokes.

19 Dental Surgery

The husband was a teetotaller, there was no other woman, and the conduct complained of was that he had drifted into the habit of winding up every meal by taking out his false teeth and hurling them at his wife.—Sir Arthur Conan Doyle

Songwriter and record producer Tony Hiller works in show business, surrounded by beautiful people with beautiful smiles. But until 1979, his own mouth was in such terrible condition that he often put his hand in front of it when he talked.

'If I tell anyone how bad my mouth was, they don't believe it. But in dental exhibitions they use pictures of my mouth before I had dental work. About eighty-five percent of my teeth had to be crowned.

'I had been thinking about having my mouth mended, but I was afraid of what might happen, and I kept putting it off. I was in Paris doing a TV show, and one of the singers said, 'Tony, your mouth looks awful.' That was the last straw. I knew I had to get something done.

'A friend of mine knew Freddie—the dentist who did the work—and introduced me to him at a party. He said that there was a lot that could be done and suggested I come to his surgery. A lot of people in my business go to Freddie; in fact to prompt a smile they'll say, 'Show me your Freddies.'

'The work took a long time because I had a bad gum problem, and they had to cut the gums. I also had a very big parting in my teeth. And the top teeth were going back and the bottom teeth protruding. Because of all the work that had to be done, it was about a year from the first time I went to Freddie's surgery until the work was finished. The

147

individual sessions were about four to five hours long.

'There were points – lots of times – when there was aggravation, especially when my gums were being cut. And there was pain when the anaesthetic wore off.

'When Freddie was working on the crowns, he gave me intravenous Valium, as well as the local anaesthetic, so I felt like I was walking on air. Of course, I had to have someone pick me up afterwards and take me home to sleep it off.

'Since I've had my teeth done, my whole life is better, even with the lads. Speaking to people is a whole new ball game.

'People say, 'Tony, you look different.' They might not be able to tell exactly what's different, but they say, 'You look great.'

'The work cost a few thousand pounds, but no sacrifice would have been too great to get the results I have.'

Open any magazine, watch any television show, and staring out from the page or screen are men and women with white, even teeth and glorious smiles. It's easy to feel inferior if your own teeth are dull or not as even as you'd like. Our teeth can be an enormous asset, but they can also be a cause of embarrassment so acute that, like Tony Hiller, you find yourself talking with your hand over your mouth.

Apart from accidents, adults lose teeth for two reasons: either decay or disease. Decay is the plague of children and young adults, but gum disease is associated with middle age. Other parts of the body repair themselves. If you break your arm and then bring the two bits into contact with one another, they will calcify together. But if you break a tooth and put the two bits together, they will never join up again.

Adults can have numerous complaints about the appearance of their teeth: there are gaps; the top teeth protrude; the teeth are misshapen or misaligned. Many people think that ugly adult teeth can't be remedied short of having them removed and replaced with dentures. Not so. Dental science is now so advanced that your mouth can be markedly improved while the roots of your teeth are kept intact. And, of course, where a tooth has been pulled, a replacement can be inserted in the blank space—an aid to both function and appearance.

Though people have started to use the term 'cosmetic dentistry', many dentists resent it. A dentist who specialises in crown work and bridge work (often described as 'cosmetic dentistry') says, 'There's no distinction between cosmetic dentistry and ordinary dentistry. I don't like the tag "cosmetic dentist", because aesthetics are integrally tied to what is healthy. What is healthy is beautiful, and what is unhealthy is often unattractive. People usually come to me with broken-down mouths. The number one thing is to get their gums healthy, remove decay, and get their whole mouth healthy. *Then* we start building up the cosmetic aspect of the mouth.'

In most cosmetic procedures there are two principals—the patient and the surgeon. In cosmetic dentistry, a third person is often involved, someone who can make all the difference to the final result: the dental technician. He or she actually makes the crown or the bridge, when that work is called for, and must be part scientist and part artist. Crowns have to fit perfectly: the roughness of a badly made crown can give the patient gingivitis, an inflammation of the gums. A dental technician's artistry comes in creating a colour and texture for the crown to match your other teeth.

Some dentists express reservations about the quality of crown and bridge work done by technicians for NHS patients compared with that done for private patients. One says, 'I feel I would be doing the patient a disservice by using crowns or bridges made for the Health Service, because they usually fit so badly and look terrible, and they often give gum problems that lead to loss of the tooth.

'For the Health Service, they make the crowns much more quickly. Technicians will quote you two charges: something like routine for Health Service crowns, or special for private crowns.'

Gaps

Gaps between teeth can sometimes be corrected. The bit of connecting membrane you have under the inner part of your lip, called the frenulum, can sometimes be very big, and fibres from that can go into the bone between the upper or lower two front teeth. Dentists can do an operation to cut that skin down by running a burr into the bone to destroy the fibres so the teeth will then come together.

Orthodontics

Most of us associate orthodontics with children, but dentists are using it increasingly to move adults' teeth. Though it takes longer for adult teeth to respond, the pressure exerted by orthodontic appliances will move the teeth into a new position. A London dentist says, 'It works very quickly provided the patient wears the appliances all the time. But some patients will only wear them at night, so it takes double the time.'

Crowns

Teeth are crowned for two reasons: to improve the appearance or to restore a tooth that is otherwise not going to survive. It may be that the filling in a tooth is so extensive that the tooth is no longer able to support itself; or it's had an abscess and somehow lost its life—the nerves are dead. Dead teeth become brittle and often discolour.

A London general-practice dentist discusses the different materials of which crowns can be made. 'Crowns at the back of the mouth have to stand up to the immense pressure of the bite, so we often put gold crowns there. Obviously, we can't put gold in the front. We can put porcelain crowns—purely china—there. Aesthetically they're the best thing short of a real tooth, but they will sometimes break.

'Now we also have bonded crowns. There you have a metal layer inside the crown; then porcelain is fired over the top, so that from the outside it looks nearly all white. Those are very much stronger than porcelain, and they've improved in appearance over the years so that now many dentists tend to use them at the front. Bonded crowns, by and large, are not going to break when you bite.'

Whatever the material, there are two basic types of crown: the jacket crown and the post crown. A London specialist describes them: 'With the jacket crown, we drill the tooth down to a stump, and then we construct a tooth in porcelain. That is cemented over the stump and fits just below the gum. When a tooth is so broken down that it has died, we are left with the root and we construct a post crown. In this procedure a gold post is cemented into the root; a jacket is then fitted over the post, and the result is a post crown.'

Bridges

A bridge, as its name implies, is an artificial tooth that spans an empty space from which another tooth has been removed. To make a bridge, the dentist will have to crown the teeth on either side. When possible, the dentist will fix the bridge permanently, but it may be necessary to put in a removeable bridge (which requires the wearer to be very conscientious in maintenance).

Consultation

The dentist who worked on Tony Hiller discusses what he does during consultations: 'First we have the hygenists clean the teeth and teach the patient how to care for them. Then we examine the gums to make sure they're in good shape. If there's a problem with the gums, we want that

151

cleared up first. There's no point in putting expensive work in a diseased foundation. Then we take photographs and X-rays to determine just what has to be done.'

Preferred Age

Dentists usually don't start crowning teeth until people are at least sixteen. One explains, 'When a tooth first erupts, the root isn't fully formed, and the nerve inside—the pulp chamber—is quite large. It begins to shrink, and by the time the patient is sixteen it probably will have shrunk sufficiently for the dentist to be able to remove the large percentage of the tooth—about half—that has to come off to permit crowning.'

Duration of Treatment

The total time treatment will take depends on the extent of the needed repairs. The number of treatments can be reduced, because anaesthetic techniques allow the dentist to work on you for four to five hours at a time without your feeling discomfort.

Anaesthesia

Dentists have available a range of anaesthesia, from simple local anaesthetic to full general anaesthetic. One London dentist says, 'The anaesthesia used depends on the procedure and the patient's wishes. What the patient wants is important, provided I get good operating conditions. Usually, when a patient is in the chair for three or four hours and I'm doing a lot of crown and bridge work, I use intravenous Valium together with a local anaesthetic and something to dry out the mouth, because saliva is a big problem in dentistry. Most patients who have the intravenous Valium say they don't feel a thing, and it's what I choose when I have work done on my own teeth.

'With the intravenous Valium and local anaesthetic,

you're very drowsy; you're not aware. You don't know that you have the local anaesthetic, because you're so sedated you don't feel it. The major work is done at the beginning, while you're heavily sedated. As you begin to come around, we're taking impressions, etc. Patients are slightly conscious during the treatment, which is a big advantage because I can get them to close their mouths, to bite, to rinse their mouths out. But a three to four-hour session seems like ten minutes to the patient.

'Patients have to be driven home by someone else; they'll have something light to eat and a few cups of coffee. They'll still be able to sleep that night and will wake up in the morning feeling fine. They may be sore for a day or two afterwards, but the pain is very slight and very easily controlled by ordinary analgesics such as codeine.'

Complications

In the hands of a competent dentist and dental technician, there is little risk of complication. Problems arise when the crown or bridge doesn't fit properly and causes gum inflammation. It may be necessary for the dentist to remove the work for the gum problem to be treated. In cases of such complication following crown work, you may lose what's left of the original tooth.

Durability of Result

No crown or bridge is going to last unless the patient takes care of it. That means using dental floss and maintaining oral hygiene. No matter how well a crown has been done, there's at least a microscopic gap where it meets the tooth, and plaque (a sticky white bacterial substance) can collect there. Some people think, 'I'll have my teeth crowned and that will be the end of my problems.' In fact, crowned teeth must receive at least as much attention as real teeth to make sure that they last.

Unfortunately, many people are given dentures before it's

153

medically necessary. When Marti Caine went to a dentist about some problems with her teeth, he said, 'Well, it's time for your dentures.' She refused and found another dentist who crowned the problem teeth. Advances in dentistry in the 1960s and 1970s have made it possible for people to have a bright smile—with their own teeth—for many years more than their parents or grandparents could.

20 Jaw Surgery

Be ... not like to horse and mule, ...
whose mouths must be held with bit and bridle,
lest they fall upon thee.
—The Book of Common Prayer

Stephen Ivers, twenty-eight, shares a small flat in Hampstead with his wife, their daughter, and two cats. He writes and directs film documentaries for an independent film organisation.

'When I came to London from York in the early seventies, I wanted to be an actor. I auditioned for one of the leading drama schools, and they accepted me. When I remember how I talked and how I looked, I can't think why.

'Not long after I began my studies, I was having a sort of counselling session with one of the staff members. He said, "One of the things we must work on straightaway is your accent; and if it's financially possible for you, I think you might consider corrective work on your jawline. You have a very long jaw, which makes you look older than you are, and the lower half of your face doesn't really suit the upper half. You'll be cast in character roles—mostly as men over forty—while you're studying here. But you'll find it difficult to get work in the commercial theatre for years and years. There are plenty of good actors who are already over forty and have years of experience."

'For years I'd been self-conscious about my overlong jaw—my top and bottom teeth didn't meet—but I didn't know that anything could be done about it. Maybe there wasn't anything that could have been done in a farming community in Yorkshire.

155

'I thought over what the counsellor had said and went back to see him two weeks later. I said that I'd like to have something done, but what? And how? He said that many people who come to the school want cosmetic work of one kind or another done before they start professional careers and that he knew of two oral surgeons in the area who did superior work. He gave me the names of both, and I picked the one whose surgery was closest to my flat.

'I knew I could afford a consultation, but I had no idea whether I could afford the surgery. When I went for an appointment, the surgeon and I had a long talk; he told me later he wanted to be sure that *I* wanted the surgery done and that I wasn't just trying to please the counsellor. I assured him that I was pleased that something could be done and that I thought it would open a whole new range of opportunities to me.

'He said that because of functional problems with my teeth not meeting, I could have the surgery done on NHS if I was willing to wait. At twenty, of course, no one wants to wait for anything.

'He told me that there's a period of four to six weeks after the operation when the jaw is in a splint. I didn't much like the sound of that, but I was determined to go through with the surgery. So we tentatively agreed that it would be scheduled during my summer break from classes.

'Just about this time my mum came down from York to visit her sister. I told them both about the surgery and what could be done. At first my mum was opposed; she said I'd inherited my father's jawline, and he'd lived with it for fifty years. I pointed out that my father was a farmer, not an actor. She finally came round, and even offered to loan me the money to have the surgery. My aunt agreed that I could stay with her after the surgery so as to be close to the surgeon in London.

'During the weeks before the surgery, there were X-rays taken and impressions of my whole mouth and chin area.

'I went into hospital the day before the operation and more tests were done. When I woke up after the surgery, I was as uncomfortable as I've ever been in my life. I had a great bandage around my head and my jaw was in a splint with my mouth all wired closed. I never had any significant pain, and I didn't require any painkillers. The surgeon said that was probably because I had a lot of swelling.

'After a week I was discharged from hospital and went to my aunt's. She had bought a liquidiser especially so she could mix up things for my liquid diet. She would pulverise meat or fish as well as fruit and vegetables. I had had no idea how many things could be turned into liquids.

'Altogether, the convalescence was nothing but a slight inconvenience. I didn't have to worry about returning to work, as I had a ten-week period before my courses resumed. After I got over feeling somewhat weak after the surgery, I helped my aunt in her garden, read, and later went into London and saw friends. The only problems were the liquid diet, which got a bit boring, and having to talk through clenched teeth. That was hard at first, but by the time the splint came off I could have made a career of gangster roles. I lost several pounds during the liquid diet regime, but I put it back on pretty quickly once I could eat solid food.

'When the splint came off and I saw my "new" face, I was surprised and pleased. It took a bit of getting used to, because it was a very big change. During the first several months, I'd catch sight of myself in a mirror and not realise I was looking at me.

'Mum cried the first time she saw me, but now she calls me "my handsome Stephen", something she could never have said before.

'During my acting studies I did get cast in a number of romantic leads—parts I'm sure the old me would never have been considered for.

'Funnily enough, in my last year of studies I decided that I really preferred writing and directing to acting. And I haven't acted since. But I'm still very pleased that I had the surgery.'

The Hapsburgs gave their name not only to an empire and

a dynasty, but also to a very distinctive jawline. A long, jutting lower jaw is often called 'a Hapsburg jaw', and it is one of the abnormal jawlines that can mar an otherwise attractive face.

The teeth and their surrounding bones and musculature play a big part in the appearance of one's face. The teeth sit in their own bit of bone, which develops at the same time as the teeth. When we're born we don't have the tooth-bearing bone; teeth and bone develop together, and the result determines the height of the face.

On the inside of the mouth, the tongue exerts its pressure outwards; on the outside, the muscles of the mouth press in the other direction; and the teeth occupy a neutral zone. The effects of imbalance of these muscles can be significant: someone with buck teeth has a soft lip musculature with no muscle tone. The muscles are not strong enough to hold the teeth in place, so they come swing outwards.

The position of teeth is usually closely related to jaw problems, which are often genetic. An oral surgeon says, 'You can inherit the Hapsburg jaw, and then your sons get it, and your daughters get it, and so on. Or perhaps you inherit your father's big teeth and your mother's small jaw. There you have another problem. Or maybe the lower jaw sticks out or recedes.'

The surgeon agrees with dentists quoted in the previous chapter that proper functioning and attractiveness are often intertwined. 'I don't regard jaw surgery as purely cosmetic surgery. In fact I don't think there's such a thing as purely cosmetic jaw or dental surgery. The whole idea is to create a better-functioning mouth as well as a better-looking one. Many patients whose teeth are in the wrong position can't eat properly. Furthermore, if they were to lose their teeth it would be very difficult to make dentures for their abnormal jaws, and they would be denture cripples for the rest of their lives. When you correct the functional abnormality, you always get an improvement in appearance.'

158

Consultation

Surgery on the jaw may be done by a plastic surgeon. More often, it is done by an oral surgeon; you may be referred by a GP or a dentist.

An oral surgeon explains the presurgical procedure: 'What we do first, after establishing motivation and expectations, is to take X-rays and work out from them whether it's the upper jaw that's too small or the lower jaw that's too large, or vice versa. Then we take impressions and photographs, we test the blood, and we make a model of the mouth. With all this information we can decide what the appropriate operation is. We have a very detailed plan for the operation before we begin it.'

If, as is usually the case, the surgery corrects a functional problem as well as a cosmetic one, the operation can be done on NHS.

Preferred Age

Sixteen is usually the minimum age at which surgeons will operate on the jaw, because its major growth has not stopped until that age. Some surgeons are wary of working on people over forty-five or fifty because of problems with bones knitting.

Hospitalisation

Expect a hospital stay of one week to ten days.

Anaesthesia

Jaw surgery is done under general anaesthetic.

Procedure

There are three different operations for the lower jaw. All three involve moving units consisting of teeth, bone, and roots with the blood supply still intact. Depending on the desired correction, the units are moved either forwards or

159

backwards in the mouth. An oral surgeon says, 'It's just carpentry, really. You lift up the gum and chisel away with the drill, slide the gum forwards or backwards into the position you want it in, and then fix it there. Sometimes we remove pieces of bone or insert a bone graft, depending on the correction we're making. Many times we must remove and/or crown teeth.

The first operation is done on a protruding lower jaw that is also too wide. Surgeons remove a wedge of teeth and gum from the front of the mouth. This allows them to bring together the remaining teeth and gums from the two sides of the mouth, resulting in a shorter, narrower jaw.

The second and third operations are to correct protruding jaws. In the second, all the surgery is done inside the mouth, so there are no external scars. By cutting the bone and moving it back, the surgeon can shorten the jaw up to one centimetre.

The third operation, which allows the surgeon to push the jaw back up to two centimetres, also involves sectioning the bone and pushing it back. But, additionally, it involves a small incision on the outside of the neck. There is a small scar in a crease line of the neck; it fades in six to nine months.

If the problem is that the upper jaw is too small, the surgeon will section off the bone in the upper jaw, pull the upper jaw forwards, and insert bone grafts in the back to hold it in place.

Depending on the complexity of the correction, the surgery takes from one to four hours.

Aftermath

To permit the bones of the jaw to knit together again, they will be immobilised in a splint, much as they would be if you had fractured your jaw. The splint will remain on for four to six weeks.

For the first forty-eight hours after surgery, you will usually have to wear an elastic pressure bandage to minimise swelling. While there is little pain associated with the operation, there is often a great deal of swelling afterwards. An oral surgeon says, 'It always looks worse than it is. You have huge swelling, but often the pain is inversely proportionate to the amount of swelling. If you've got a big swelling, often there's hardly any pain at all. If you don't get swelling, you may have pain. No one seems to know why.'

Convalescence

For the first month or two, you will probably visit the surgeon twice a week so that the progress of your healing can be checked.

During the time you have the splint on, you'll be on a liquid or semi-liquid diet. Everything will be put in a liquidiser, and you'll drink it through a straw. Fortunately, even with a full set of teeth there's a gap into which a straw will fit. (If you've been trying to lose a few pounds, this surgery may help; oral surgeons report that their patients almost invariably lose weight during the time the splint is on.)

If you're really keen to get back to work, you can usually return after three weeks. You'll still have a good deal of swelling, as well as the splint, but that shouldn't interfere too much with your efficiency in most lines of work. Should you prefer to stay off the job until the splint is removed, count on four to six weeks' absence.

When deciding how much time to take off work, you might consider how much talking you have to do on the job. You'll be able to talk even though your teeth are wired together, but you may have some problems being understood on the telephone. One oral surgeon says people adapt very quickly. 'They may sound a bit like George Raft at first, but in a very short time they become surprisingly adept at talking without moving their teeth.'

If you have reason to be unhappy with your jawline, you can be thankful that the human jaw isn't set in marble. It can be manoeuvered and manipulated by a skilful surgeon so that the appearance of the face is improved—along with the functions of the jaws and teeth.

161

21 Breast Surgery

How do you like them? Like a pear, a lemon,
à la Montgolfiere, half an apple, or a cantaloup?
Go on, choose, don't be embarrassed ...
—Colette

Over the last half century or so, fashions in breast size have changed. In the twenties flappers bound their breasts, and since then fashion has favoured either the well-endowed Marilyn Monroe style or the more angular, flat-chested look of Twiggy.

Sometimes women are dissatisfied with their natural breasts and wish to have them enlarged or reduced in size. In other cases, women lose one or both breasts in surgery to treat breast cancer; many such women want to replace a semblance of what disease has taken and so opt for breast reconstruction after mastectomy.

Techniques for breast augmentation, reduction, and restoration improve continually, but none of the procedures is yet without its drawbacks.

Breast Augmentation

Kay Locke is a native of Canterbury, where she still lives and works as a secretary. She was thirty-three and married, the mother of three, when she decided to have cosmetic surgery to enlarge her breasts. Her experience was unfortunate.

'I guess I had the operation done from sexual vanity. My husband liked big-breasted women. Even though I'm

162

thin, I had big breasts before the children were born. Then they disappeared. The only place I have stretch marks is on my bust, because that's where I lost the weight.

'I had no trouble with the operation. I went in that morning and came home the next day. There was very little scarring; you can just see it underneath my breast. It had faded within the first two weeks.

'There was a lot of itching at first, but I had no problem with any of the things you're supposed to have difficulty doing—peeling potatoes, making beds, or driving.

'The trouble I've had with them is that they're painful, and the left one is terribly hard. I have to keep going back to the surgeon. He gets rid of the hardness by squeezing the breast, which is very painful.

'My husband didn't like the feel of them. I can understand why. When I press up against someone, I feel sure that I've got two bricks or two tennis balls in there and that they can feel them.

'Now, since my husband and I have separated, I'm afraid to go to bed with anybody because of the pain when they're touched. My breasts feel artificial to me, and it's a cheat.'

Celia Stone is a forty-four-year-old solicitor who practises in London; her husband is a barrister. They live with their two teenaged daughters in Weybridge, Surrey. Celia Stone didn't lose her breasts after pregnancy; she had hardly any to start with. But at the age of forty-two and after two children, she had a successful augmentation operation and is very pleased with the results.

'I first became conscious of my problem as soon as I realised that other girls had breasts and I hadn't. It was difficult to get clothes to fit because I was out of proportion to the sizes in which they make dresses.

'It's a problem you learn to live with, and I can't say that it worried me particularly.

'But it's nice not to have to worry about whether your padding is slipping. When I told my husband I wanted to have the operation, he said, "I like you as you are." But I wanted to have it done for me, if for nobody else.

163

'I'm very close to our family doctor. When I approached her about it, she reassured me that there was nothing wrong with me, but she referred me to a cosmetic surgeon. He said he could do what I wanted, which was to make me the size I was with my padded bra.

'I didn't want anyone but my husband to know, so I told my daughters I was going in for a D and C.

'I went into hospital the morning of the operation and was in for two nights afterwards. That was a few years ago, and I understand hospital stays are shorter now. I had a general anaesthetic and no pain or discomfort. When it was over, I was all strapped up and felt like a mummy. A week later, I went back to see the surgeon, and he took all the binding off. Then I wore a bra day and night for six weeks.

'I've still got scars. Unfortunately, I'm one of those people who scar. The scars went lumpy, so the surgeon gave me an injection that softened them up. They're still there, but they've faded.

'I didn't want to make a fuss afterwards, so I just carried on as normal, but for the first three weeks I did no heavy work. I couldn't do anything strenuous or anything where I had to put my arms over my head, like hanging out the washing. I was told I shouldn't drive, but I did. I drove my husband's car, which has power steering, and I didn't go far. When I had to go to a garden show a little distance away, I persuaded a friend to drive. I told her I had cracked my ribs.

'One of the breasts went rather hard, but the surgeon popped it, and it's been all right since.

'I feel as though the breasts are me. They're firmer than average. Of course, I don't know what real breasts feel like. I don't think about them anymore. Well, every once in a while I look at them, and they're pretty nice.

'Having the surgery was a real boost for me. I gained more confidence, and I feel better. I can wear bikinis and dresses with tiny straps. I couldn't have worn them before, when I had to wear a bra with everything.

'It was something I did for me. It just depends on how you want to spend money. If I'd had a choice of having a fur coat or having my breasts done, I'd have had the operation—and I did.'

Women who seek breast augmentation are sometimes those who were born with very little breast tissue and who have spent their lives envying their more buxom sisters. Other women have lost breast tissue as an aftermath of childbirth.

Whatever the reason a woman may feel her breast size is inadequate, surgery is the only method of enlarging breasts. All the creams—hormonal or otherwise—won't help; even exercise won't do it, because there are very few voluntary muscles in the breast (a voluntary muscle can be strengthened by exercise).

Breast augmentation surgery, whose technical name is augmentation mammaplasty, is a relatively simple procedure, and the results when the surgery is properly done appear natural and are not easily detectable. As with other cosmetic procedures, there can be complications that lead patients to be unhappy with the results of their surgery.

Surgeons say that they are especially careful in choosing patients for breast augmentation, because a woman might be attributing other problems to the size of her breasts. One psychiatrist says, 'Some women have marital problems. They say, "He doesn't like me because I don't have big enough breasts. He thinks I'm masculine." Other women have had children; during pregnancy their breasts were bigger, and they feel their husbands paid more attention to them.'

The best motive for the operation, psychiatrists and plastic surgeons agree, is simple vanity. As Celia Stone said, 'It was something I did for me.'

Plastic surgeons say that most requests for breast augmentation come from women between the ages of thirty-five and forty-five who have had one or more children and lost breast tissue.

Breast augmentation will not affect your ability to breastfeed, should you have a child after the surgery. The operation will not interfere with detection of breast

165

cancer, nor has it ever been associated in any way with the development of breast cancer.

One caution: don't let anyone inject liquid silicone into your breasts. This was a popular method of breast augmentation some years ago, but there were sometimes disastrous results when the silicone travelled to other parts of the body and caused serious medical problems. Liquid silicone has been banned from use in surgery in the United States, but some surgeons in Britain and other countries continue to use it for such other surgical procedures as filling out wrinkles. (Liquid silicone *injections* into the breasts should not be confused with the silicone gel *implants* used safely in augmentation surgery.)

Consultation

What the surgeon will be doing in a breast augmentation operation is to put inside your body a 'falsie' that should be as soft and pliable as your own breast.

In deciding how much to augment your breasts, you and the surgeon will have to take into consideration your height, weight, and general figure type. The surgeon won't be able to transform Audrey Hepburn into Sophia Loren, because an Audrey Hepburn figure won't have enough skin to cover such a large implant without undue tension in the skin and blood vessels. If the desired results can't be achieved in a first operation, a second one to augment the augmentation can be performed after the skin has stretched sufficiently to handle a larger implant.

The search for satisfactory implants for undersized breasts began in the 1930s with the injection of paraffin into the breasts and continued with the use of Teflon sponges. Neither method was satisfactory. For a time, injections of liquid silicone seemed to be the answer, but the results were catastrophic. Not only did the liquid silicone prevent detection of breast cancer, but it left the breast and moved throughout the body.

Currently, the prosthesis, or implant, most often used is a round, soft silicone capsule filled with silicone jel. The capsules come in a variety of sizes. Another style of implant is like an empty silicone balloon when inserted; after it is in place, the surgeon fills it with saline solution through a tube, which is sealed and then trimmed off before the surgeon stitches the wound. The balloons require a smaller incision and can be filled with as little or as much solution needed to make the breasts match in size.

Breast augmentation usually cannot be done on NHS.

Preferred Age

The operation can be done on anyone over eighteen or twenty years of age. There is no upper age limit for a healthy person.

Hospitalisation

Again, this will depend largely on the individual (age, general health) and the anaesthetic you choose. With local anaesthetic you can usually go home within twenty-four hours of the operation. With general anaesthetic you'll probably be in hospital for about two days.

Anaesthesia

Opinion is divided among surgeons. Most prefer general anaesthetic, but say that the operation can be done under a local anaesthetic if costs of anaesthetist and hospital are prohibitively expensive for the patient.

Procedure

In the most commonly used procedure, which takes about one hour to perform, the surgeon makes an incision about two inches long in the skin fold below the breast (inframammary fold). This creates a pocket, into which the prosthesis is then inserted, between the breast tissue and the chest wall. Your natural breast is in front of the prosthesis.

An alternative technique involves a semicircular incision around the areola (the pigmented area at the nipple), starting about halfway down the areola and going around its bottom. This technique is less commonly used, because it's harder for the surgeon to get the implant in; the advantage is that the scar is virtually undetectable.

In another technique designed to minimise the scars from breast augmentation, the prostheses are inserted through tiny horizontal slits in the armpits and then moved inside the body to the breasts. This technique hides the scar in the armpit, but, because of the distance from the incision to the breast, the operation is more difficult. A plasic surgeon reports that the American surgeon who devised this technique has abandoned it because he has encountered too many problems with bleeding.

Aftermath

After the operation you'll have bandages around your chest for twenty-four to forty-eight hours. Celia Stone says, 'It doesn't hurt. It's like a tight bra pulling on your ribs.' But she felt very listless for the first twenty-four hours after the operation. 'Not even my two favourites, Sean Connery and Robin Ellis, could have stirred any enthusiasm in me.'

Both surgeons and patients agree that there is no post-operative pain, though you may experience a stiffness in the breasts for a time after the surgery. If you exert yourself too soon, you will feel a pulling in the stitches.

There will probably be post-operative swelling for ten days to two weeks. For a few weeks after the surgery, there may be bruising and stiffness around the breast and shoulders.

As soon as the dressings are removed, you'll begin to wear a bra night and day for about four weeks; surgeons also advise that you sleep on your back.

Convalescence

After six weeks your new breasts can be touched, so you can then resume a normal sex life—but gently.

Most surgeons want you to restrict other activities for the first two to three months after the operation. You should avoid any tasks that require raising your arms over your head—such as lifting things from shelves—or any movements involving the shoulder muscles. A surgeon explains that such restrictions are advisable because movement involving the shoulder muscles affects the chest muscles. In the last few years, some surgeons have become less strict on these restraints than they used to be, but still want you to avoid really strenuous activities, such as tennis and swimming, for three weeks to a month.

Some surgeons prefer that you not drive for a few weeks after the surgery because you may pull on the stitches while shifting gears.

After healing, the implants should feel supple and natural.

Scars

For the most common type implant procedure, the incision is in the fold under the breast and so the tiny semicircular scar is hidden by the breast. After it fades in a few months, you should be the only one to know it was there.

In the second, or 'balloon', method, there is a tiny scar at the edge of the areola; when that fades it will be virtually invisible.

Complications

Most surgeons agree that breast augmentation is far easier than breast reduction from the surgeon's point of view, but often much lower in patient satisfaction. The reason for patients' disappointments is usually that a hardness develops in the implant area. (Some surgeons believe that daily massaging helps to prevent such a development.)

Our bodies aren't happy when a foreign substance is introduced into them, and they may well gear up to resist the invader. In these cases a thick, fibrous capsule forms around the implant. (Surgeons estimate that this happens in twenty to thirty per cent of breast augmentation patients.) As Kay Locke said, the implant feels like a brick and becomes very uncomfortable. The usual remedy is for the surgeon to stand behind you and squeeze the breast until the scarlike capsule around the implant 'pops'. This procedure works in most cases, though it may have to be repeated. In very few cases, the prosthesis must be surgically removed; a replacement may be implanted later, if the patient wishes to go through it all again.

Writer Yvonne Dunleavy of the New York *Post* reports that some Amercian doctors have stopped doing breast augmentation operations because they find the incidence of the fibrous capsule formations unacceptably high.

As with all surgery, there's the possibility of haematoma (collection of blood under the skin) and infection. If the haematoma is serious enough, the surgeon may have to operate; in some cases, the problem can lead to loss of the implant.

While a certain amount of post-operative depression is common after any surgery, plastic surgeons say that they notice a greater tendency to depression in women who have had breast augmentation. You may feel very depressed, and the slightest provocation may make you cry. Try not to worry—it's a 'normal' reaction and usually lasts for only a few weeks.

Most women who have had breast augmentation say that they feel the same sensations when their 'new' breasts are touched as they did before surgery. But many also say that their augmented breasts rarely feel the same *to* the touch as normal breasts. In fact surgeons report that the most common complaint they get after breast augmentation surgery is about the texture or hardness of the new breasts.

Durability of Result

The results of breast augmentation surgery are permanent. Breast augmentation requires judicious consideration before it's undertaken. You may have the good luck not to have the complication of a fibrous capsule formation; but if you are unlucky enough to have that problem develop, it can be—as it was (and is) for Kay Locke—a serious psychological problem.

Breast Reduction

It's been a year and a half since forty-three-year-old Caitlin Williams underwent surgery for breast reduction. She and her family live in Aberystwyth, where she and her husband operate a small restaurant in an area frequented by tourists.

'I had my second child when I was thirty. Until then I was very slim and wore a 34B bra. A few months after my daughter was born, my breasts started growing and growing and became abnormally large. I thought I must be gaining weight, but every other part of my body had returned to the size it was before I was pregnant. Sometimes this condition comes on teenage girls, but it came to me after childbirth. I finally went to a size 44D bra.

'It was terrible. My shoulders used to bleed where the bra straps cut them, even though I had my bras specially made with padding in the straps. I developed bursitis and couldn't lift my arms.

'I used to sweat under my breasts and get an odour there. I'd take three or four baths a day. I'd also get infections, apparently caused by the sweating, which had to be cleared up with salves.

'As you can imagine, I was also very self-conscious about my appearance. It was bad enough when our regular customers came in, because I knew that they had seen this great change in me. But the tourist season was almost unbearable; the customers didn't look at *me*—they looked at my chest.

171

'All my clothes had to be specially made, because I wore a size eight bottom and a size forty-six top.

'I'd see my gynaecologist twice a year, and I'd cry at every visit. He said that there was an operation he could do, but that I would lose the nipple and end up with a stub.

'My mother had had breast cancer, and every time she heard I was thinking of having an operation on my breasts, she said she'd never talk to me if I did such a thing. My husband was also against it at first because he thought it would hurt me.

'I told him that I was very, very unhappy and that the condition was abnormal, and he came round. He wasn't happy, but at least he was neutral. But my mother wouldn't budge. She was shocked that I'd have an operation I didn't need, and she also somehow thought it might cause breast cancer. Finally I asked my gynaecologist to talk to her. He calmed her fears and explained that the operation was really for my health. She still wasn't happy about it, but she no longer threatened to stop speaking to me.

'Finally I just decided, "They're not going through what I am. It's my life, and I've got to do it." So I told the gynaecologist I would go through with the operation, though I knew I'd lose the nipples.

'Three days before the operation, my gynaecologist called me. He said, "I just can't do that operation on you. You're too young. I want you to see a plastic surgeon." He recommended a plastic surgeon who then did the breast reduction operation on me.

'I had a two-hour consultation with him before the surgery. The operation took over four hours, and he took out fourteen pounds of fat. He removed my nipples and put them in a solution and then stitched them back at the end of the operation.

'When I woke, I was wearing a compression bandage from the waist to shoulders. I felt as though I couldn't breathe. The bandages were on for two or three days.

'I was supposed to leave hospital after a week. The day before I was to leave, I developed a fever of 104° and the surgeon discovered that I had a staph infection. Instead of

172

being in hospital one week, I was there over ten weeks.

'The surgeon who operated on me has referred several women to me who are interested in the surgery but who haven't made up their minds. At first he said he didn't know if he should refer them because of my complication with the infection, which I probably got in the operating theatre. I told him that even with the infection and all I went through because of it, I'd still have the operation done again.

'It was very important to me that the operation doesn't interfere with detection of breast cancer. I have a breast check-up every four months, not because of my operation but because of my mother's cancer. It was fortunate that I'd had my children before I had the surgery, because you can't breastfeed afterwards.

'I can't tell you how happy it makes me to walk into a department store and buy a bra, a blouse, or a dress after years of having everything made.

'I'm lucky that I didn't lose sensation in my breasts; they feel completely normal. After about a year the scars faded, and they're now barely visible.'

Women with small breasts often wish that they were built like their more generously endowed sisters, but many women who wear 42D bras would gladly change places with one who wears a 32A. However unhappy flat-chested women feel about their state, it doesn't cause a health problem, nor does it cause them to be regarded as grotesque.

Caitlin Williams recalls that the occupant of the bed next to her when she had her breast reduction surgery was a seventeen-year-old girl who was having the same operation. 'She hadn't been to school for two years. Her breasts were so enormous that she couldn't sit or stand straight; she kept falling forward. She wouldn't go out, so her family had to have a tutor come to the house.'

Women with over-large breasts are not only the objects of stares; they also have health problems. They often experience rashes, bleeding, and problems in posture. And their breast size is very limiting in choice of clothing—most have no choice but to wear loose overblouses. Such leisure activities as tennis and jogging are made difficult or impossible by their breast size.

Many surgeons who specialise in breast surgery say that breast augmentation is an easier operation for the surgeon but that breast reduction is much higher in patient satisfaction, because it helps patients to lead a normal life again. It makes a great change aesthetically—and, often, an even bigger change in the patient's feeling of well-being.

A caution: if you're contemplating breast surgery, it's especially important to involve your spouse, because of emphatic personal feelings he may have had about such surgery. The American weekly magazine *Parade* reported this story about a German couple:

> Monika Rau, 42, owner of a boutique in Nuremberg, West Germany, had a bust equal to her age. For years men would look at her in awe and wonderment, but Monika was embarrassed, and her too-large bosom made the wearing of stylish clothes impossible. Several weeks ago when her husband, salesman Hans Joerge, left on a business trip, Monika called on a plastic surgeon and submitted to a three-hour operation which reduced her bust size by eight inches.
>
> When her husband returned and saw his newly dimensional wife, he grew furious. 'You have no right to alter your body without my permission!' he shouted. He stomped out of the house, drove to his lawyer, and asked the lawyer to file a divorce suit on his behalf.

Consultation

Surgeons want to be sure that you're aware of the serious nature of this surgery. As one says, 'It's a difficult operation because I have to take the breast apart, reshape it, and then drape the skin over the new breast.

'Patients must be aware that there are usually quite a few scars. I don't like to do the operation on women under

174

thirty-five because the scars are inclined to get thicker and red.

'I also want to be sure that a woman who might be thinking of having children knows that she won't be able to breastfeed after the operation.'

Surgeons want you to be as close as possible to your ideal weight—it's far safer for any operation. In breast reduction, your body weight can also affect the result. A surgeon says, 'Since part of the breast is fat, you'll change the shape of the breast and its size if you lose weight after the operation. That might make you think you could reduce the size of large breasts by losing weight, but that isn't true. You can lose six or seven stone, and your breasts may get a little smaller, but if you have the typical large breasts, they just don't reduce in size.'

The same surgeon goes on: 'I want to be sure the patient knows that there are two things I can't promise: that the new breasts are going to be a certain, predetermined, size; that the reduced breasts are going to match exactly in size. No two breasts are exactly the same size to begin with, so it's hard to achieve that in the operation.'

Your surgeon may ask that you donate blood before the surgery. There can be a fair amount of blood loss during the operation, because it involves vascular tissue. A blood transfusion usually isn't necessary, but many surgeons like to have the patient's own blood available as a precaution.

Breast reduction can very often be done on NHS.

Preferred Age

There are some disagreements among surgeons about suitable ages for breast reduction. Many prefer to work on patients between sixteen and twenty years old. Others prefer women who have finished child-bearing, because of the loss of ability to breastfeed. One surgeon says, 'I won't look at anyone over forty,' but others have operated on patients as old as seventy-two. Those who operate on older patients say that physical fitness is more important than chronological age.

175

Hospitalisation

Because breast reduction is major surgery, there is a hospital stay involved. The length varies according to the condition of the patient and the philosophy of the individual surgeon. One says that he usually keeps his patients in hospital for only two days. 'I put in catheters to drain out any accumulation of fluid; they come out after two days and then the patient can go home.' Other surgeons prefer longer hospital stays, sometimes up to a week.

Anaesthesia

Breast reduction is done under general anaesthetic.

Procedure

With a surgical marking pen, surgeons usually draw on your breasts the planned lines for the incisions. Some do this after the anaesthesia has been administered; others prefer to do it while you are still sitting up.

The two most common procedures in breast surgery differ mainly in the treatment of the nipple area.

In the pedicle technique, the nipple remains attached to a thread of skin, thus preserving the blood supply to it. When the surgeon finishes removing fat and breast tissue, he or she attaches the nipple to its new location. This technique doesn't result in as much loss of sensation as the free-nipple graft, but it limits the amount of breast tissue that can be removed.

The free-nipple graft is usually done on women who have really gigantic breasts or on older women for whom the reduction in breast size is of such value that it offsets the loss of sensation in the nipple area. In this procedure the surgeon removes the nipple-areolar complex (the nipple and its surrounding dark skin), puts it in a solution, reduces the breast, and reattaches the nipple-areolar complex. 'The problem,' says a surgeon, 'is that it always looks like it's been pasted back on—it somehow doesn't look real.'

176

The operation takes a minimum of two hours.

Aftermath

After the surgery you'll either be wrapped in sterile gauze dressings or wearing a bra specially tailored for breast reduction patients. Patients generally agree that there isn't much pain associated with the operation after the first twenty-four hours. A surgeon explains that breast reduction is relatively pain free because 'everything is on the surface. It's not like either operating on the abdomen, where you cut through muscle, or going into the chest between ribs.'

The stitches will begin to come out about five days after the operation, and all should be removed by the end of twenty-one days.

Convalescence

After you're discharged from hospital, there will be a period of about three weeks before recovery, and during that time your activities will be restricted. For the first ten days or so, you won't be able to bathe. During the three-week recovery period there's to be no reaching, no shoulder movements that cause the chest muscles to move, and no sports like tennis or golf. For about a month after the operation, you'll wear a bra both day and night.

It takes up to a year for the breast to settle into its new position.

Scars

There is scarring from the breast reduction operation: around the nipple-areolar complex, down the front of the breast, and along the fold under the breast. A plastic surgeon describes the scar as 'an inverted T with a keyhole at the top.' It will fade in about a year, though some women experience better fading than others. In some, the scars continue to be clearly visible, and a few women even

177

develop the raised, reddened scars known as keloids.

Complications

Because nerves have been severed, there's often decreased sensation in the nipple-areolar complex; in some cases, sensation returns over a period of time.

Besides the risks common to all surgery, on rare occasions the breast operation leads to the loss of the nipple-areolar complex. It can slough off if the blood supply is lost. The cause may be a technical error during the surgery, or an infection compromising the blood supply. However, surgeons say that such a problem is very uncommon if the surgery is performed correctly. If the nipple-areolar complex is lost, a new one can be fashioned of skin taken from the genital area.

Breast Reduction
in Males

Some males develop breasts, especially during puberty. Usually the breasts disappear; but when they persist, they're a source of great embarrassment, especially for young men who want to engage in sports.

Such breasts present no health problem, but they can be removed surgically to solve the psychological problems they so often cause. The surgeon makes the incision around the nipple-areolar complex or in the fold under the breast. The nipple is not disturbed.

For centuries, women with over-large breasts had no recourse but to suffer in silence. Their flat-chested sisters had the remedy (unsatisfactory though it often was) of wearing artificial padding, but women with exceedingly large breasts had no relief for their physical and psychological pain. Fortunately, the techniques of modernday cosmetic surgery allow women with this problem to return to normality.

Breast Uplift

Drooping breasts—the shift of the mass of the breast from top to bottom—can follow pregnancy or can be an early sign of middle age. Producing a large elastic from his desk, a plastic surgeon explained the problem. 'Imagine that you suspended a weight from this elastic,' he said. 'For a while the elastic would support the weight nicely, but eventually the law of gravity would take over and the weight would stretch the elastic. That's what happens to breasts when they start sagging with middle age.

'The sagging has to do with the breast's supporting structure, which has stretched through age, pregnancy, or, sometimes, weight loss. In other words, there's too much skin for the breast. The breast skin forms a sort of natural brassiere, supporting the breast tissue. Sometimes nature's brassiere "gives out", just as the manufactured kind does.

'Through surgery we can restore the breast envelope that has stretched. The incision is similar to that for breast reduction, but we don't remove tissue. We rewrap the skin and make it a sling and support for the breast.

'Sometimes, especially after pregnancy, when breasts have not only sagged but also become smaller, we put in an implant to give the breasts shape. But you can't cure sagging with augmentation alone. In fact that would aggravate the condition, because the weight of the implant would just make the breasts sag more.

'The operation is done under general anaesthesia. There is a hospital stay of approximately two days, and the scars will be the same as those after breast reduction, with the same attendant problems.

'I usually have patients wear a special support bra for at least a month, sometimes for several months.

'I've found that patients are usually very pleased with

179

the results of this operation. Their morale is raised as well as their breasts!'

Breast Asymmetry Correction

Although no one's breasts are exactly alike, the difference is usually not noticeable and so doesn't cause a problem.

However, some women's breasts differ markedly from each other in size, a condition that can lead to psychological problems as well as to the more mundane difficulty of finding bras and clothing that fit. Linda West, thirty-seven, explains her situation: 'Have you ever bent down wearing a bra-type top and had to wonder whether your breast would pop out because one side of the bra was too large? Or laid back in the sun with your bra still in perfect shape but your breasts spreading themselves out like pancakes up to the chin and under the arm?' Linda West had always had one breast larger than the other. Now, after cosmetic surgery, her breasts are separate, full, and the same size.

Asymmetrical breasts may be normal but for their widely varying sizes; or they may be some combination of normal/very small/very large.

Using the techniques of augmentation and reduction, surgeons can go a long way to correcting asymmetrical breasts. Sometimes surgery is required on only one breast; in other cases, it's necessary to augment one breast and reduce the other.

Breast Reconstruction after Mastectomy

In early 1979 Brenda James was told that the lump found in her breast was malignant and that she would have to undergo a mastectomy. Even though she was sixty-three, she decided that she would have breast reconstruction surgery after the mastectomy.

'Having had two lumps removed from my breasts over the years, both benign, I had asked my doctor in two annual checkups to order a mammography for me. He said he didn't believe in doing that. I finally told him that I was going to change GPs; he then ordered the mammography, and it showed another lump. The biopsy showed it to be malignant, and I was scheduled for a modified radical mastectomy.

'Because of my history of breast problems, I had read widely about what can be done, and I thought breast reconstuction after mastectomy was a wonderful idea and that if I ever did develop breast cancer, I would definitely have reconstruction.

'I told the surgeon that I would like a plastic surgeon to be involved in the operation so that incisions would be the best kind for future reconstruction. At first he refused. Then he phoned me a day later and said he had changed his mind, that if it was so important to my morale, he would permit it even though he wasn't pleased about it.

'The plastic surgeon rotated a flap from my abdomen up to my breast (it was still attached at the naval) and another flap was rotated from my back and brought around to the front. The two flaps covered the area where breast tissue and skin had been removed.

'The plastic surgeon had asked me if I wanted him to save the nipple; he said that he could attach it to my thigh until I was ready for the reconstruction. I told him that I didn't really care about the nipple; what I wanted from the reconstruction was the shape of the breast.

181

'I had a great deal of pain after the mastectomy, probably because I'd had the flap procedure done as well. I had only a little discomfort after the actual reconstruction.

'As it happened, I changed plastic surgeons, because I had been so unhappy with the hospital where I'd had the mastectomy. A surgeon who'd operated on my husband for a heart problem recommended another plastic surgeon to me. I was very impressed with him at the consultation, because he explained everything very thoroughly. He emphasised that although the reconstructed breast would not look like the other breast, it would allow me to wear normal bras and eliminate any embarrassment in wearing clothes.

'He told me I'd be in hospital for three or four days; in fact, I stayed five.

'The surgery was done ten months after the mastectomy. Afterwards I had a binding dressing that stayed on for two days; then the surgeon put a lighter dressing on.

'I went to his surgery a few days after I came home and he took out some of the stitches. When I went back again, I brought a bra. When he took the dressing off, I put the bra on, and I wore it night and day for several weeks.

'The implant was hard at first, but it softened up over nine months. I got a numbness sometimes in my upper chest and underarm area. It wasn't constant—it would come and go. The surgeon said that a nerve had been nicked in either the mastectomy or during the reconstruction. The numbness ended after a year or so.

'The peculiar thing was that the breast that had been reconstructed was hot for the first six months. I told the surgeon, and he said he couldn't explain it.

'I didn't keep the operation a secret from anyone. Many people looked at me as though I had taken leave of my senses. I found that many people are insensitive to other people's problems.

'As for me, I feel wonderful. I'm whole again.'

About most of the operations discussed in this book, there is a fair consensus among surgeons as to when and whether they should be done; but there exists a mass of disagreement about breast restoration after mastectomy. Surgeon A said he was unsure whether the reconstruction was justified at all because of the even minor risk of reactivating the cancer. Surgeon B said reconstruction could be done, but six to nine months should elapse after the mastectomy. And Surgeon C said reconstruction could often be done during the same operation in which the cancerous breast is removed.

Many of his fellows find Surgeon A's position conservative, in the negative sense of that term.

The argument against surgeon C's position is presented by Surgeon B: 'The complications of mastectomy are real enough in terms of wound healing. I'm not sure that I would want to superimpose the potential complications of breast reconstruction.' He prefers to wait to see the area healed, past its initial scar reaction, and softening and maturing before doing the reconstruction.'

A woman has to face myriad problems when she or a doctor finds a lump in her breast. The most serious question, of course, is what treatment will be undertaken if the lump proves to be cancerous. For many years the standard treatment was the very mutilating radical mastectomy: it not only removed the breast and lympth nodes, but also left a great hollow under the clavicle on removal of the pectoral muscles, which pass from the ribs to the upper arms on each side of the chest.

Surgeons now more commonly use the modified radical mastectomy: they remove the breast and generally also remove some or all lymph nodes, but leave the pectoral muscles intact. (Sometimes a skin graft is necessary to close the wound in either a radical or modified radical mastectomy.)

A third technique has gained increasing popularity in the last few years: the lumpectomy—removal of the cancerous lump and some surrounding tissue—followed by radiation therapy.

A fourth procedure, the subcutaneous mastectomy, involves only the removal of the fatty tissue of the breast. This operation is preventative . It is designed not for women who *have* cancer, but for those at higher-than-

183

average *risk* of developing breast cancer. A woman with a pronounced family history of breast cancer or one with especially dense breasts (which develop small cysts and make it difficult to diagnose a cancer by either X-ray or clinical examination) may be advised to undergo a subcutaneous mastectomy to spare herself years of anguish and repeated biopsies.

Many women are unaware that after most radical, modified, or subcutaneous mastectomies, they can have plastic surgery for breast restoration. Though surgeons can't restore the breast to its premastectomy appearance, they can make it possible for a woman to feel comfortable in a variety of clothes, such as bathing suits and evening gowns, that would be awkward to wear otherwise. Psychologically the reconstruction can be an enormous boost for a woman who has spent months or even years looking at a flat area where her breast used to be.

One patient wrote to her surgeon after undergoing successful reconstruction. 'I don't have to use a lot of padding anymore. Maybe I'll use a little padding to match the other breast, but I can wear my bra. I can wear a two-piece bathing suit. When I take a shower, it isn't a totally flat area; there's something there. When I get undressed at night, *there's something there.*'

While the physical distress is great for patients of any age, the psychological suffering is usually increased in younger patients. A plastic surgeon recalls, 'I had one patient of sixty. She and her husband had been together for thirty-two years, and she knew he meant it when he said he loved her far more than her breasts. She had reconstruction primarily because it was a big help in enabling her to wear the kinds of clothes she wanted to. I had another woman of about thirty. She was really beautiful and had a terrific figure, and it was obvious that her body image was an important element in her relationships with other people. She too had the restoration surgery. When she came in to see me about six months later, she told me that she and her boyfriend had broken off. I don't know how much a part of that break-up was caused by the breast problems.'

Just as plastic surgeons differ among themselves on the issue of breast reconstruction, so also do the general surgeons who prefer mastectomies. Some are supportive and understanding. Others feel that the patient should be grateful to be alive and cancer free and should not be concerned about such trivial vanities (in their estimation) as reconstruction. Fortunately, the latter attitude seems less prevalent than it used to be, as increased recognition is given to the role women should play in making decisions about breast-cancer surgery and its aftermath.

Consultation

The consultation may take place before the mastectomy or after it. Patients have had restoration as long as twenty years after mastectomy.

If before mastectomy, the plastic surgeon can confer with the general surgeon about the shape of the incision and the scar from the mastectomy. One plastic surgeon said, 'When we're asked beforehand by general surgeons, we would probably like to see the scar made in a transverse [horizontal] direction—if they can do their surgery adequately through a transverse incision, which they can most of the time. That gives us the opportunity to do a reconstruction in which scars will be in the least noticeable area, so that they might not show even in the tiniest of bathing suits. A vertical scar may go all the way up the shoulder, and that's hard to camouflage in a bathing suit or an evening gown.

On the other hand, a woman may have just had a mastectomy and, after seeing herself minus a breast, may ask the general surgeon what can be done. The general surgeon may then ask a plastic surgeon to see her while she's recuperating in hospital. The plastic surgeon won't be performing the operation at that time, but he or she can probably give the patient an idea of what can be done.

As always, surgeons want to be sure that your expectations match the probable results. In this case they are especially careful, since the mastectomy itself is such a psychological trauma. A plastic surgeon says, 'The

185

patient must understand that I can't restore a breast that looks just like the one she lost. Sometimes a reconstructed breast doesn't look very good at all. That doesn't mean it's a bad *surgical* result; but if the surgeon is faced with limitations in the case itself, the result is limited. I also make clear that there usually won't be any sensation in the restored breast, because most of the sensory nerves in the area will have been destroyed.

'Curiously, I find that between the mastectomy and the time I am scheduled to do the reconstruction several months later, many women change their minds and don't want the operation. Some women adjust to an exterior breast prosthesis during that time and decide against further surgery. Some say they want reconstruction of the breast as well as an artificial nipple—which is done in a separate procedure. Often after the restoration of the shape of the breast, they decide they don't care about the nipple.'

In an effort to make the two breasts as close in size as possible, surgeons sometimes recommend the reduction of the remaining breast.

Breast reconstruction can be done on NHS.

Hospitalisation

The length of the hospital stay can range from overnight to six or seven days, depending on the complexity of the procedure (see below).

Anaesthesia

The operation requires general anaesthetic.

Procedure

The site and shape of the incision for reconstruction depend on the mastectomy incision. The surgeon must make the new incision so as not to compromise the blood supply to the area—which could happen if the new incision is too close to the old one. Usually the surgeon will make the incision either in the crease under the breast or in the side of the breast. The incision itself is small—about an inch and a half to two inches long—and is placed so that it will be camouflaged even in a skimpy bathing suit.

The simplest reconstruction is made possible when the mastectomy has left a lot of soft tissue and the skin is relatively loose and stretchable. The operation is then much the same as a breast augmentation: the implant, which is the same as those used in breast augmentations, is put under the remaining fatty tissue. Sometimes the surgeon moves muscle up (if muscle remains after the mastectomy) to give a little more soft-tissue coverage in the area.

The reconstruction is somewhat more complicated in patients who do not have adequate soft-tissue coverage. There may have been a skin graft to close the wound made during the mastectomy, or there may have been scarring after radiation. Since the skin is tight, it won't accommodate an implant, and tissue must be brought in from somewhere else. Some surgeons 'mobilise' some abdominal and fatty tissue and slide it upwards. That provides slack, and an implant can be inserted under it. (Sometimes it's necessary to put a graft on the abdomen to make up for the loss of tissue there.)

Another way a surgeon may solve the problem of limited soft tissue is to put in an implant not as large as the patient would ultimately like to have. With the passage of time, the skin may give and stretch, and then a larger implant can be put in. Alternatively, patients might be given implants that can be gradually increased in size by injections of saline into them.

A relatively new technique to solve the problem of limited soft tissue is described by a plastic surgeon: 'One of the techniques developed over the past few years is what we call a myocutaneous flap. We take part of the latissimas dorsi—the big muscle that attaches behind the shoulder and runs down the side. We can take an island of skin and leave it attached to part of the muscle, free that part of the muscle, and rotate the skin and muscle over to the breast as a flap. That adds both skin and muscle to the breast area to give more bulk. Under that we can put an implant.

'We're sure to tell the patient beforehand that with this technique we will produce a scar where we take the island of tissue. There's a minimal functional problem in using that muscle. There's no interference with back movement, and the patient can still do pretty much everything she'd want to do.'

If the patient wants the nipple reconstructed as well as the breast, the surgeon usually waits a month or more and then does it on an outpatient basis. Surgeons delay doing this procedure, because they want to be sure that healing is proceeding well, without infection. Surgeons are also concerned about circulation, and the reconstructed nipple depends for survival on good circulation in the skin. The reconstructed nipple is made from skin taken either from the pigmented area of the other nipple or from the genital area. Some surgeons even raise the centre part of the reconstructed nipple so that it looks as nearly like a real nipple as possible.

The time of the procedure varies according to the work being done. The simple placement of an implant takes about one hour, whereas moving a flap into the area may take three hours or more.

Aftermath

For the first few days after the surgery, you will probably be wearing a soft bandage to give support in the breast area. The dressing is soft so that there won't be excessive pressure on the area that could compromise the blood circulation.

Depending on the extent of the surgery, the surgeon may or may not use a drain afterwards. If there is expected to be serum and blood, often the surgeon will put in a suction catheter for a day or two.

There will be bruising, which will probably persist for about two weeks.

The amount of pain will depend on how much muscle

has been involved in the surgery. If the surgeon has not dealt with muscle (there may no longer be muscle there), then it's much less painful than if the pectoral muscle has been lifted up to place the implant under it. (The reason an appendectomy is so painful for a day or two afterwards is that muscles have been stretched.) If muscle has been involved, there will be two or three days of pain, during which the surgeon will prescribe narcotics or other painkillers.

Convalescence

After you're discharged from the hospital, the surgeon will probably want to see you at his or her consulting rooms in about three days to see that the dressing doesn't bind and that there isn't any pressure in the area.

Although there are special bras made to be worn after the operation, one surgeon believes they just add to the cost. 'I tell the patient to come to my rooms with a very soft bra without seams so that we can use that as our supportive dressing. I instruct her to wear it at all times, even when sleeping, for about two weeks. After that, she can take it off when she sleeps.'

The same surgeon cautions his patients that they won't ever be able to wear ribbed or wired bras, a precaution to prevent blood circulation problems. He might permit it for an occasional special event for which you would want to wear an evening gown, but he doesn't want pressure placed on the area of the reconstruction.

The stitches come out in about a week; then you can shower and bathe normally.

You'll be asked to be relatively quiet for the first two weeks, avoiding shoulder movement when possible and keeping your arms at your sides. After about two weeks you can begin to resume some normal activities. One surgeon says, 'I tell patients after two weeks to let their comfort be their guide. If they feel too much stretching and pulling, they should be a little gentle. After three weeks to a month, I have them begin to resume doing everything they want to do. I tell them that in playing

189

tennis or undertaking an activity like it, at first there may well be stretching, pulling, and aches. That's because there's scar tissue and it has to stretch, but probably no harm is being done to the wound area after that length of time.'

Scars

The scar from the actual insertion of the implant is similar to the scar after breast augmentation. However, if skin flaps or grafts are used, there will be additional scars; their location and size will depend on the size of the flap or graft and the area in which it is used.

Complications

Surgeons say that the complications from reconstruction are similar to those from the mastectomy. There may be bleeding in the pocket that's been created for the implant, in which case the surgeon will probably have to operate again to eliminate the bleeding. There may be a delay in a healing of the wound. There may be compromised circulation to the skin followed by sloughing of part of the skin. If that occurs, the surgeon may have to remove the implant. Postoperative infection may also cause the surgeon to remove the implant. Though the implant, as an inert substance, doesn't cause reaction in the body, if there is infection around it, then it reacts more like a foreign body and the surgeon must remove it in order for the infection to clear.

If the implant has to be removed, that does not mean that the reconstruction process can't be repeated and the implant reinserted.

Durability of Result

The results of breast reconstruction are permanent.

Breast reconstruction certainly isn't perfect and may be needed less and less as surgeons adopt less mutilating methods of treating breast cancer. Until then, reconstruction offers hope of return to something close to normality for women who have suffered the trauma of mastectomy.

22 Body Surgery

The Queen was in her chamber, and she was middling old,
Her petticoat was satin, and her stomacher was gold.
Backwards and forwards and sideways did she pass,
Making up her mind to face the cruel looking-glass.
—Rudyard Kipling

In a time when long dresses covered a woman's lower body, who could tell if her abdomen showed evidence of several pregnancies or if her buttocks were drooping? She had no worries about how she'd look in a bikini or in tight blue jeans.

As the twentieth century has progressed, women have worn fewer and fewer clothes in public. They've also become more and more self-conscious about their appearance in revealing clothing. In increasing numbers, women are turning to plastic surgeons to sculpt their bodies into more pleasing shapes.

Of the operations discussed in this chapter, only the one on the abdomen is generally accepted by surgeons. Many prefer not to do thigh and buttock lifts or operations on bat arms because the scars can be worse, in terms of comfort and/or appearance, than the condition that the surgical procedure is performed to correct. One surgeon says, 'I warn patients about the scars, but I still find they often resent them when it's too late.'

Abdominal Skin Tightening

Lisa Newgard, thirty-eight, and her husband live in Dartmouth, where they own and operate a boat chartering business. She recently underwent surgery to remove stretch marks from her abdomen.

'I had three pregnancies between the time I was twenty-five and thirty-five. Each time I gained three stone, and lost all but about five pounds after the birth.

'We spend most of our time around people who are physically fit, and I was upset at how I looked. I finally managed to diet off the fifteen or twenty pounds I'd gained, but I still had the stretch marks as well as all sorts of loose skin on my lower abdomen.

'Through some connections he'd made in his business, my husband Mark was able to arrange a holiday in Marbella, Spain, for about half of what it would otherwise have cost. He told me about it at Christmas, and the holiday was set for May.

'I knew that I couldn't go onto a beach in a bikini; of course, that's not the end of the world, but it motivated me to take action.

'I first went to my GP and asked her to prescribe a programme of exercises that would get me in shape by May. She gave me the bad news that exercise may do wonders for muscles but does nothing for the excess skin. And neither does dieting. She said that the only option was plastic surgery. I knew that I'd have to go some distance to have it done; I chose London because my parents live there. My GP recommended a surgeon there, and I phoned and made an appointment for the following week.

'At the consultation he examined me and asked me all sorts of questions; he said later he wanted to be sure I didn't think I was going to get back the figure I had when I was eighteen.

193

'After he told me what he could and couldn't do, he said that I should go home and think it over—I would be subjecting myself to major surgery—and call if I decided I wanted to go through with it.

'I had told my husband that I wanted the surgery and why; he made a few jokes about my wanting to pick up some rich yacht-owner, but didn't say much else. I must confess I didn't tell him some of the things the surgeon told me—about not being able to stand upright for a few days, for example.

'After a week was up, I called the surgeon, and he set the surgery for the end of March, which meant that I would have almost two months to recuperate before we left for Spain.

'I went up to London a few days before the surgery; the children stayed at home with my husband. I went into hospital the day before the surgery. They did some tests; I took a sleeping pill and went to sleep.

'The morning of the surgery, the surgeon came in and drew lines on my stomach with a great black marking pencil. He said these were the lines for the incisions, and he wanted to draw them while I was standing up. He also said my pubic hair would be shaved before the operation.

'The first few days after the operation were hateful. I was lying in bed with my knees up; the first time I tried to move I was hit by this wave of pain. That made me not want to move at all. Finally, the surgeon insisted that I try to get out of bed. It hurt, but it was also funny. I had to walk stooped over, and I felt I looked like a monkey.

'When I left hospital, I stayed with my parents for about two weeks. It took that long before I could walk comfortably upright. Fortunately, I had nothing to do and didn't need to move around a lot.

'After I returned home, I tried not to do anything that required lifting or stretching.

'I was quite well by the time we went to Marbella, and I had a lovely time. The scar was nicely hidden in my bikini.

'Altogether it was a very difficult experience. It's hard to say whether I'd do it again, knowing what I now know. I

194

like having a flat tummy, but it was quite an ordeal.'

Motherhood has many joys, but one of them is not the stretch marks that most women have on their abdomens after pregnancy. And, whether or not it is associated with pregnancy, the loss of a great deal of weight can produce a sense of fitness and accomplishment—and abdominal skin that is hanging and flabby.

In both cases the contents of the abdomen have stretched the abdominal skin, which has a limited ability to retract elastically. An operation called an abdominoplasty (or sometimes a lipectomy) is designed to tighten the abdominal area after the excess weight has been lost.

Many people mistakenly believe that this operation allows them to lose weight without submitting to the rigours of a diet. Not true: in fact responsible surgeons insist that patients remain stable at or close to their ideal body weight for a period of time before they will consider performing the surgery.

Consultation

A plastic surgeon describes how he evaluates patients who come to him for abdominoplasty: 'There are two criteria, the physical and the psychological. For this operation, the physical criteria are secondary. I'm interested in the patients' expectations and their intelligence and common sense, because I have to judge how responsible they are going to be in following the postoperative regimen, which is very important to a good result.

'Physically, I want patients who are at a proper weight for their size. It's important that their weight be stable, because weight gain or loss after the surgery simply sabotages the effect of the operation. I want patients who have a significant excess of abdominal skin, and whose stretch marks, if that's the reason for the operation, are located on a horizontal line below the top of the naval.

'In the operation we pull down the skin above the navel and sew it to the skin in the pubic area, after trimming off the skin that was below the navel. The area of skin I remove is a triangle, with the apex at the top of the navel and the sides extending outwards and downwards to the hips. Stretch marks above the navel will move down, but they won't be excised.

'I prefer patients with no previous surgical scars on the abdomen. Such scars make it more difficult to get an acceptable flap of abdominal skin and fatty tissues.

'The ideal candidate is a woman in her twenties, thirties, or early forties who has postpartum redundancy [superfluous or excess skin] but who is athletic and has taken care of herself. I also prefer someone who is through with childbearing, because if she has a child after this surgery, she'll have the same problem again.

'It's important for patients to know that this is major surgery involving a hospital stay of several days, a period of convalescence at home, and a substantial scar, which can take up to a year to settle and even then probably won't be invisible. One unfortunate thing about this operation is that the scars tend to be other than hairline thin. No surgeon would reasonably promise a patient such a scar, but the scar can usually be hidden in the confines of normal clothing.

'Some surgeons ask at the consultation that patients bring to the hospital a bathing-suit bottom or the panties they usually wear, so that the surgeon can mark the line just before the operation and can try to hide the scar so it won't be visible in a brief undergarment or bikini.'

Surgeons will often ask that you provide some of your own blood during the weeks before the surgery. There is considerable blood loss during this operation, and most surgeons prefer to use the patient's own blood, should a transfusion be necessary.

In cases in which an abdominoplasty corrects a functional problem (for example, an apron of skin that hangs so far that it interferes with urination), it can be done on NHS.

Hospitalisation

The hospital stay is four to ten days. During the first few days there will be substantial discomfort or pain, and you won't be even moderately comfortable walking for at least four or five days.

Anaesthesia

The operation is done under general anaesthetic.

Procedure

Before the surgery, some surgeons will put you on a liquid diet and will give enemas and laxatives so that you won't have a bowel movement for some time after surgery. This prevents strain on the muscles and stitches in the area of the operation.

On the operating table you will be bent, with back slightly raised and knees flexed.

The pubic hair will be shaved to make it easier for the surgeon to make the incision. (Some surgeons have you shave yourself before you enter the hospital.)

A large incision is made across the lower abdomen. There are different varieties in the shape of the incision, which in turn will, of course, determine the shape of the scar. The surgeon decides which incision to use on the basis of personal preference for a certain technique and the specifics of the patient's problem.

The surgeon raises a large flap of skin, subcutaneous tissue, and fat off the underlying abdominal wall musculature and then separates the skin of the raised flap from the underlying tissue, going from the level of the lower abdomen (the pubic bone) to that of the rib cage. The navel is raised, but is left attached to its underlying blood supply. Your knees-flexed position on the operating table aids the surgeon in pulling down the flap of skin; the excess is trimmed off. The surgeon also tightens vertical muscles in the abdomen with sutures, to make the waistline appear slightly smaller. Then the navel is put back—although it is now poking through a new hole, one

197

made in skin that used to be above the navel.

The opertion takes two hours or more. A plastic surgeon says, 'The time depends on the quality of the surgeon's assistance [the number of assistants and their levels of experience and expertise], how much the patient weighs, and how much bleeding the surgeon encounters.'

Aftermath

Surgeons have different approaches to bandaging after the operation. Some put on a light dressing and an elastic binder with mild compression. Others user a plaster cast. Their choice depends on how much pressure they feel is necessary to support the area of the surgery.

The head and foot of your hospital bed will be raised so that your position will be as close as possible to that on the operating table. As the days pass, the position of the bed—and you—will become more nearly horizontal.

Especially for the first few days, there will be a good deal of pain, particularly when you attempt to move. Most of the pain comes from the sutures used to bring the muscles back into position. Surgeons prescribe appropriate painkillers.

There will also be noticeable swelling and discoloration around the abdominal flap. The time it takes for the swelling to subside varies. For most people it takes about three weeks, but surgeons report cases in which the swelling has lasted five to six weeks. The discoloration disappears within about three weeks.

A plastic surgeon reports, 'I usually try to get patients out of bed the day after the operation. Occasionally I wait until the second day. I don't want them lying in bed for a prolonged time, because of the dangers of phlebitis and lung problems.

'At first they can't stand upright. That takes from several days to a couple of weeks, depending on how much I've trimmed. Another consideration is the willingness of the patient to attempt to stand. Some people resist doing so because of the discomfort associated with it. There's little the surgeon can do about that. Patients must supervise themselves and be their own taskmasters.'

Convalescence

The stitches come out ten to fourteen days following surgery. The length of time you must be off work will depend on your surgeon and on what type of work you do. Some surgeons want all patients to be off work for four to eight weeks. Others take into consideration the nature of your job. Someone with a desk job would probably be at home ten days to two weeks (after five days in hospital) and could probably then go back to work. Someone who does heavy physical work would have to be at home an additional two to four weeks before returning to work.

At home, surgeons want you to avoid heavy physical exertion including housework—for four to six weeks, sometimes even longer. If you don't, a surgeon explains, 'The physical exertion could cause haemorrhaging under the flap. In a few cases the exertion may not be voluntary. I had one patient who developed a violent cough shortly after she got home, and that tore the sutures.'

During your convalescence, many surgeons want you to sit with knees up for at least ten days, to use a pillow under your knees when you sleep, and to avoid wearing tight clothing over the area operated on.

You will progressively become more active, and the surgeon may prescribe a programme of graded exercises, such as walks. The amount of pain and discomfort connected with motion is variable. Some patients are pain free, within a limited scope of activity, after two weeks. Most have completely recovered in six weeks.

Complications

Three possible complications of abdominoplasty are similar to those from other types of surgery: haemorrhage, infection, and skin slough (the falling off of dead skin).

As with some other surgery, there can be the problem of temporary or lasting numbness—in this case, around the upper part of the leg. Surgeons try to avoid cutting the

199

nerve that promotes skin sensitivity in that area, but it infrequently happens that the nerve is cut.

Another problem could be necrosis (death) of the navel. Surgeons try to avoid this complication by meticulous dissection in the navel area so that they don't divide the blood supply. If necrosis occurs and the navel tissue is destroyed (a rare event), there are techniques that can be used to create the impression of a navel.

Thigh and Buttock Lifts

The thigh lift and the buttock lift are very often done as a single operation. The buttock lift, or 'bottom lift', is designed to take care of very large, overhanging, or sagging buttocks. An operation on the outside of the thigh can remove so-called 'riding breeches', pads of fat that make a woman look as though she's wearing a riding costume. Operating on the inside of the thigh is intended to take care of flabby, hanging skin caused by weight loss or age.

A plastic surgeon summarises the reasons that he and many of his colleagues are reluctant to do thigh and buttock lifts. 'The operation was developed in South America, where the women are built differently, and their fat is distributed differently.' Another problem is that the scars, which are large, tend to 'drift' with the passage of time, and they drift downwards. A scar that's hidden under a bathing suit shortly after the operation will have migrated in a few years down to the leg.

'There's also an increased risk of infection associated with thigh and buttock lifts, because you're operating in the dirtiest area of the body. And operations are more difficult as you get into the legs, because there's poor drainage in areas below the heart, and poor blood supply.'

Thigh and buttock lifts are entirely cosmetic operations and cannot be done on NHS.

Hospitalisation

The hospital stay lasts from four to six days.

Anaesthesia

The surgery is done under general anaesthetic.

Procedure

The operations are very similar. For the inner-thigh operation, the surgeon simply extends the incisions made for the riding breeches/buttocks operation.

Before the operation the surgeon will usually draw the incision line while you are standing.

During the surgery you will be lying face down on the operating table.

The two horizontal incisions start in the inner portion of the thigh; they come around towards the back and diverge at the buttocks—one incision going above the crease and the other below it—and move to the outside of the thigh towards the hipbone.

To correct the riding breeches deformity, fat is not actually removed from the body; it is simply moved nearer the buttocks. To decrease the size of the buttocks, the surgeon removes both skin and fat. The buttocks will have a rounder contour because sagging skin has been removed, but gravity will pull the skin down again.

To conclude the operation, the surgeon joins the two incision lines and stitches them together so that they are positioned in the crease below the buttocks.

To tighten loose skin on the inside of the thigh, the surgeon makes an incision in the fold where the trunk and the thigh join (the inguinal fold); the excess skin is pulled up and removed and the incision closed.

Operations on the buttocks and thighs can take up to four hours.

Aftermath

You will be lying in much the same position after thigh and buttock lifts as after an abdominoplasty, with knees flexed. As with the other operation, the surgeon will try to get you up the day after the operation or the one following to avoid the possibility of phlebitis or lung problems.

Convalescence

When you go home, you'll have the same restrictions on physical exertion that you'd have after an abdomino-plasty. After buttock/thigh surgery, you won't be able to sit—only to walk or lie down—for two or three weeks. Sitting strains the stitches and is also painful.

Complications

Other than the usual complications that may occur after surgery, patients who have thigh/buttock lifts may find that their legs swell after the surgery; and sometimes, if the stitches have too much tension, there may be stretching of the vagina. The most serious possible complication is phlebitis (inflammation of a vein).

Bat-arms Correction

Either weight loss or ageing can lead to the development of bat arms, characterised by loose, hanging flesh on the upper arms. People with this condition are often embarrassed to be seen with arms uncovered.

In the past, surgeons have done a procedure in which they make an elliptical incision along the length of the upper arm and remove the excess skin. However, most surgeons do not perform this procedure any longer in any but the most extreme cases. The scars from the surgery are so bad, they say, that the patient must still conceal the area under long sleeves, so the operation doesn't free them to wear the clothes they'd like.

A possible complication of this operation is damage to the nerves of the arm or forearm, resulting in either numbness or a burning sensation around the scar (both effects often permanent), which makes the area so sensitive that it can't bear the weight of even light clothing.

In the long history of plastic surgery, body surgery is the newest chapter. Many plastic surgeons flatly refuse to perform these operations, with the exception of the abdominoplasty, because of the severity of the resultant scars and the possible complications.

23 The Sexual You

How do I love thee?—Elizabeth Barrett Browning

Countless books, ever more detailed and explicit, have been written on the hows and whys of love and sex. It's not surprising, then, that many of us, in all our newfound sophistication, feel we don't measure up to some current standard of sexuality or physical allure. Sometimes, though, our problems go beyond attitudes and appearances and are more directly related to a real or perceived disorder of sexual function. Such problems may range from the relatively simple one of vaginal slackness to the more disturbing one of male impotence.

Vaginal Repair

Usually after they have had several children, some women complain about a loss of sensation in the vagina and ask to have the vaginal passage narrowed so that they and their partners can again achieve the sexual satisfaction they once enjoyed. Other women—whether their vaginal dimensions are average or greater than average, altered or unaltered by childbirth—simply seek to better the fit of a partner's relatively narrow penis.

The surgery is also done to correct medical problems caused by a bulging of the bladder or rectum into the vagina.

204

Vaginal repair is done not by a plastic surgeon, but by a gynaecologist; in fact, it *should* be done only by a gynaecologist. Someone who is not well familiar with the operation can cause dysfunction by overnarrowing the opening.

Consultation

After an examination, you and the gynaecologist will discuss how much you would like the vaginal opening altered. Usually it's possible to make it any size you want.

However, gynaecologists are especially careful about the selection of patients for this operation, because they want to be sure that you're not hoping for more than the operation can deliver. One gynaecologist estimates that as many as fifty percent of the patients requesting this operation have 'some sexual hang-up in their background, or a marital problem they hope the operation will cure. It's very important to weed those people out.'

If the operation corrects a medical problem of the vagina, it can be done on NHS.

Preferred Age

Your age is much less important than your childbearing plans. Surgeons want to be sure that you don't plan to have more children after undergoing vaginal repair. The surgery may interfere with the vagina's ability to stretch enough to accommodate a normal delivery, so a Caesarean section would be necessary.

Hospitalisation

Depending on your surgeon (and perhaps on your bank balance), you can expect to be in hospital at least overnight, but it's more likely that you'll be in three days or more.

205

Anaesthesia

The operation is done under general anaesthetic.

Procedure

The surgeon opens the front and back walls of the vagina and shortens and tightens the supporting ligaments and muscles to narrow the vaginal opening.

The operation takes about one hour.

Because the incisions are made inside the vagina, there are no scars.

Aftermath

According to a gynaecologist, 'There's a certain amount of discomfort—in fact, pain—involved in tightening the perineal muscles, because the area where it's done—between the vagina and the rectum—is very sensitive.'

Sometimes there is difficulty urinating during the first few days, so a catheter (a tube for withdrawing liquids) may be placed in the bladder.

Convalescence

For three to four days, keep up and about, because you'll find sitting uncomfortable. Bed-rest is also uncomfortable, but it's better than sitting.

There may be occasional slight bleeding for several weeks.

You should be able to resume sexual intercourse in six to eight weeks.

Penile Implants

Most men suffer from impotence at some point in their lives, often during time of worry or stress. But for some men the period of impotence doesn't end, and each failed attempt at sex increases the anxiety.

Psychiatrists say that the origin of most impotence is psychological. Physicians differ on whether or not to operate on such patients if extended psychotherapy has not been effective. Some surgeons believe that operating for a psychological problem is not justifiable; others say that successful surgery can help the psychological situation.

With a minority of men suffering from impotence, the cause is organic, most frequently diabetes or vascular disease, or a combination of the two; some men also suffer from a low hormone level. Some urologists will consider implants for such patients.

Consultation

A urologist says, 'For a man, his sexuality and his virility have a great deal to do with his self-concept. A man cannot fake an erection. When a man suffers impotence, it takes a long time for him to admit the problem, even to himself. Often, the problem develops over a period of time. The man gets an erection, but it's not firm, or it goes down just as he is about to enter the woman.

'When a patient is referred for treatment for impotence, we do extensive testing. We evaluate their hormones and learn as much as we can about them both physically and psychologically. We always involve a psychiatrist, because impotence may be one symptom of a pervasive problem.

'If the cause turns out to be organic, many men are very relieved. Most cases of organic impotence are found in older men, but there are some in young men as well.

'If, after several interviews with a psychiatrist and several more with me, we and the patient decide that the

207

cause is organic and that a prosthesis will do something positive for the man, we will decide to go ahead with surgery.

'I treated one man recently who had been married for twenty-one years. He had diabetes and was not able to work. He received some small pension, but his wife had become the principal breadwinner in the family. His impotence was organic—caused by the diabetes—but it was causing him a psychological problem in that he felt he'd completely lost control of his life. In fact he was considering leaving his wife and children. He had little sensation in his penis before the surgery, and, of course, he doesn't have any more now, but he has a better attitude because he feels that he's satisfying his wife.

'We now have a choice of implants. One consists of two silicone rods inserted into the penis. The penis is rigid and always erect, it is held next to the body with jockey shorts. Recently a variation on this prosthesis has been introduced that allows for greater flexibility in bending the penis.

'The other type of prosthesis is inflatable, a silicone rubber balloon type supplied with a reservoir and a pump. The man pumps a valve and fluid goes into the penis and makes it erect; he releases a valve and the fluid returns to the reservoir. This type comes closest to simulating a real erection, because the penis starts as flaccid and grows hard. But there have also been more complications with it.

'The type of prosthesis is the patient's choice. The rubber silicone is less expensive than the inflatable prosthesis, which involves a system of connections and valves. The choice often depends on whether the man could tolerate having an erect penis all the time and how he feels he'll look to his sexual partner.

'Whatever function the man had before the surgery, he will have afterwards. For example, if the canal for semen has not been blocked, he will still be able to ejaculate.

'Like most of my colleagues, I will operate only on men whose impotence has an organic cause, and, I insist on extensive psychiatric evaluations and therapy.'

Preferred Age

Age is not a factor in determining whether to perform the surgery.

Hospitalisation

The period of hospitalisation is usually seven to ten days.

Anaesthesia

The operation is done under general anaesthetic.

Procedure

For the rigid prosthesis, an incision about one inch long is made in the pubic hair. The two silicone rods are inserted in the shaft of the penis.

For the inflatable implant, the incision is made just above the penis. The urologist inserts two inflatable cylinders attached to a fluid-containing reservoir in the lower abdomen. The reservoir is connected to a pump in the scrotum near the testes.

The surgery takes about two hours.

Aftermath

There is both soreness and swelling, sometimes severe, in the area of the surgery.

Convalescence

Most patients must be off work for at least two weeks. The degree of discomfort after the surgery varies. Sometimes it's painful to have the prosthesis rubbing against the body, and sometimes the area is too sensitive for jockey shorts to be worn. The pain can last for two months or more.

Sexual relations can be resumed six to eight weeks after the operation.

Complications

Complications fall into two groups, physical and psychological. Physically, there is the possibility of infection; or there is the persistence of pain that sometimes leads to the patient asking that the prosthesis be removed.

With the inflatable prosthesis, there is the additional complication of leakage of fluid from the reservoir.

There are also possible psychological complications. A psychiatrist says, 'Before the surgery, the men were often interested in sex, but unable to perform. After the surgery, they can have an erection at will but are sometimes less interested in sex. In normal sex, the erection is a "reward" that comes after love play. But when a man has an erection at all times, the love play isn't really necessary, and the satisfaction sometimes decreases for both the man and his sexual partner.'

24 Scar Revision

Be fond of the man who jests at his scars,
if you like; but never believe he is being
on the level with you.
—Pamela Hansford Johnson

Edith Taylor is a thirty-one-year-old nurse. She and her husband live in Guilford, Surrey. In February, 1977, they were returning from a visit to her sister in Rye when a passing car forced the Taylors' car off the road and into a ditch. Edith was thrown through the windscreen and her face was badly cut.

'I don't remember anything, of course. I was taken to a small local hospital, where the young man in the emergency room did his best to stitch together the cuts on my face. For the first few days I was so happy to be alive and not to be blind or to have lost a limb that I didn't think much about the scars. I also had bandages on my face, so I really didn't know what had happened.

'I'd always had fair, smooth skin. When I first saw it with the scars—well, I didn't look like a gargoyle, exactly, but there were several nasty scars on different parts of my face.

'I work for a paediatrician, and I overheard several children in his surgery ask their mothers questions about me. I felt sorry for the mothers, who were very embarrassed.

'About two months after the accident—when I was still wearing large sunglasses whenever possible—I went to our family doctor and asked him what I could have done about the scars. I didn't really fancy living with that face for the rest of my life.

211

'Our GP sent me to a plastic surgeon in London, who said I could have the surgery done on the NHS if I was willing to wait; or I could have it done privately. I talked to my husband, who had only minor bruises from the accident, and he agreed that we would use part of our savings so that I could have the operation done privately as soon as possible.

'When I saw the plastic surgeon about nine months after the accident, he said the scars had settled and healed enough so that he could work on them. Shortly afterwards I went to hospital for the first operation. Altogether there were three operations, and I was in hospital just one night for each of them. I was lucky that no skin grafts were involved.

'The first operation was the most extensive, and the most difficult for me. When it was over I had a large bandage on my face, and for a few days it was difficult for me to move my mouth to speak or eat. I lived mostly on cream soups, which I drank through a straw.

'After each of the operations I was home for about a week, though I'm sure I could have gone back to work earlier after the second and third. I scheduled one operation during my own holidays, one during my employer's, and one just before a bank holiday, so I really missed little work.

'Where I had several large, ugly scars, I now have very fine scars; if I'm wearing make up, you can't tell they are there unless you know beforehand.

'Naturally I'm very pleased at the difference. I think I'm as happy for my husband as for myself; I'm sure that every time he looked at my face, he felt terribly guilty. The accident wasn't his fault, but I'm sure he accused himself of my disfigurement and is very happy that the signs of it are now minimal.'

This chapter is titled 'Scar Revision' rather than 'Scar Removal' because it is impossible to remove or completely eliminate a scar. Scars are Nature's method of healing wounds. What plastic surgery can do is to replace an ugly, disfiguring scar with a less conspicuous one.

The most important surgery for repairing a scar usually takes place in the initial treatment, before the scar has even formed. When the cause of a scar is a laceration, the patient is often brought to the emergency room of a nearby hospital and is completely dependent on the skills of the attending physician or surgeon. If the hospital is in an urban area, it is sometimes possible to get a plastic surgeon to come and do the initial operation. But often, because of time of day or hospital location, it isn't possible to wait for a plastic surgeon to arrive and the emergency room staff must do their best. Understandably, they lack the skills of experienced plastic surgeons; and they are under pressure to work quickly to save the patient's life and health.

For burn victims in particular, many general surgeons try to involve a plastic surgeon in the treatment as early as possible; in some cases a plastic surgeon directs the care from the outset.

With burns, as with lacerations, the depth is important. Everyone has experienced a thermal burn—a superficial burn caused by, say, splashing very hot water on the skin. The body responds to the irritation with a slight inflammation (simply an increased blood supply to an area). When healing is complete, the inflammation goes away; the area doesn't need the extra blood supply anymore.

If the water is hotter and is left on longer, there's a deeper injury to the skin—a partial-thickness burn. It's usually marked by the formation of blisters, because the outer layer of the skin hasn't just been damaged; it's been killed. The dead skin separates from the live skin underneath and fluid collects between the layers.

In the most serious burns, such as those that can be suffered in a house fire, the full thickness of the skin is killed—from the epidermis all the way through the dermis, down to the subcutaneous fat. The skin is completely mummified. In cases of such full-thickness burns, surgeons put on a skin graft; that can cut down tremendously on contracture, one of the major problems with burns and their resultant scars. Contracture is a formation of thick, fibrous tissues that prevents adjacent muscles, tendons, and joints from performing their proper functions. For example, a person who suffered a burn in the neck area under the chin might be unable to raise the chin because of contracture.

Consultation

Plastic surgeons are interested in the location of the scars, their cause, and their stage in the healing process. It takes six to twelve months before a scar matures: if it's red, it's still healing. Often the passage of time will make surgery unnecessary because the scar has faded to an acceptable colour. Scars are most easily repaired in certain locations —firm sites such as forehead and nose—as opposed to areas, such as the cheeks, where the tissue is more mobile. Semicircular or U-shaped scars are the most difficult to revise.

A plastic surgeon summarises his considerations in the revision of a facial scar: 'We look first at how the scar may have affected the form of the face. The second thing our eye seeks is symmetry: is one side of the face the same as the other? Next, how does the colour match between the scarred area and the normal skin? The last thing we note is the texture. Skin in different areas has different texture.'

In the consultation the surgeon will consider the amount of skin available to stretch, the blood supply, and the elasticity of your skin. As one gets older and the skin loses its elasticity, scar revision is often more successful.

Surgeons are often consulted about hypertrophic or keloid scars. A hypertrophic scar is an enlarged scar that keeps growing for up to three months after surgery and then gradually softens. Children are more prone than adults to such scars. A keloid is a hypertrophic scar that extends beyond the margins of the original injury and tends to recur after being excised. People of various racial groups have a greater tendency to keloids. The lowest tendency is among whites of fair complexion. Blacks have a much higher tendency to keloids, as do Orientals, especially Japanese.

Because there is such a wide variety of scars—as there is of causes of scars—the surgeon will present a plan based on your individual needs. In some cases skin grafts will be needed; in others, not. Sometimes only a single surgical procedure is necessary or useful; sometimes a series of procedures will yield better results.

A plastic surgeon says, 'We try to stress that once an injury has healed by a scar, there's no way that the injury can be undone. After that, we emphasise the positive in that there is almost always something that can be done to improve the appearance of the scar. Usually the worse the scar, the more we can do to improve it.'

Hospitalisation

The period of hospitalisation varies with the complexity of the procedures. Some minor scar revisions are done on an outpatient basis; but when the scars are larger, or for the first (usually the major) revision in a series, often there is a hospital stay varying from overnight to several days.

Anaesthesia

Most procedures are done under general anaesthetic, but some simpler procedures (for example, the last and the least extensive in a series) may be done under local anaesthetic.

Procedure

In the simplest operation, the surgeon cuts out the scar, separates the skin on both sides from the tissues underneath, and then stitches together the edges of the healthy skin.

If the scar is larger, the surgeon may have to use a 'local flap'—a partly detached mass of skin and tissue that has its own blood supply and is adjacent to the scar. Local flaps are effective because they are the same type of skin and are from the same area of the body; they give the best match of

215

colour and symmetry because they have the same amount of subcutaneous fat.

If the scarred area is very large, the surgeon will use a skin graft. For example, for a facial scar, surgeons may graft skin from in front of or behind the ear, or from the back of the neck.

When revising a keloid, the surgeon cuts out the scar and a small area of skin around it. The edges of the skin are stitched together, and, to help prevent the keloid from recurring, the new scar is injected with a steroid.

When scar revision is done by a skilled plastic surgeon, a fine, hairline, scar often replaces a large, ugly scar. In making the incision for scar revision, some surgeons use a technique known as Z-plasty; the Z describes the shape of the incision, a shape employed to take tension off the healing wound so it doesn't pull apart.

Aftermath

Because procedures differ so, the healing process varies widely in the amount of pain afterwards (and therefore the type of painkilling drugs necessary) and in the extent of bandaging. After major scar-revision surgery on the face, you may, like Edith Taylor, have to subsist on a liquid diet for a few days because of the bandages.

If bleeding has been properly controlled during the surgery, there should be little bruising or swelling.

Convalescence

After the revision of a small scar, you can return to normal activities very quickly, often within a week of leaving the hospital. If the procedure has been more extensive, surgeons usually suggest that you stay home for at least a week after your hospital discharge and rest, relax, and eat well to promote healing. Surgeons sometimes prescribe vitamins during this period.

Following scar revision on the body, you should limit such activities as stretching. After surgery on the face, avoid excessive movements of the facial muscles.

216

Complications

Surgery to revise scars carries with it the same complications as other surgery: a collection of blood under the skin, infection, and skin slough.

Pioneering work in scar revision was done by Sir Archibald McIndoe who treated pilots and other airmen who were badly burned in the Battle of Britain. Techniques developed by McIndoe and others continue to help restore the appearance of those disfigured by accidents or burns.

Afterword

Consider beauty a sufficient end ...—W. B. Yeats

If you decide to visit another country for the first time, you look for a good travel guide—one that removes the fear of the unknown, points out the attractions of the place, and warns of pitfalls to be considered.

Appearances was designed to be such a guide to a territory unfamiliar to most of us—cosmetic surgery. After consulting many experts in the field, I have tried to present a balanced perspective: to point out that cosmetic surgery has both its positive and negative aspects. Just as a holiday can leave us feeling relaxed and refreshed, so cosmetic surgery can lead to an improved self-image. But, like any surgery, it can lead to complications and, in some cases, to disappointment with the results.

Like any responsible guide, *Appearances* is not trying to sell you on a trip as the answer to all your problems. It simply arms you with plenty of information if you embark on the journey to a new appearance.

ELIZABETH DEVINE

219

Appendix: Costs

Some people believe that cosmetic surgery done at commercial clinics will be less expensive than that done privately by a surgeon; this is often not true. An experienced consultant plastic surgeon looked at a brochure from a clinic in the London area and said, 'A woman could have four face lifts from me for the price of one at this clinic.' Below are sample costs for surgeons' fees for various cosmetic procedures. They represent a range considered legitimate and fair by most hospital-affiliated surgeons in the U.K. Surgeons' fees vary considerably, depending on the experience of the surgeon, the area of the country, and the complexity of the operation. The additional costs a patient will incur will be: anaesthetist's fee (if general anaesthetic is used), rental of the operating theatre, drugs and dressings, cost of hospital stay (where applicable). Costs shown were correct as of January 1, 1982.

abdomen lift	£500-£650
bat ears	£250-£350
breast augmentation	£500-£650
breast reconstruction after mastectomy	£650-£800
breast reduction	£650-£700
chemical skin peel	£200-£250
chin implant	£175-£250
dermabrasion	£200-£300
electrolysis	£3.50-£5 per fifteen minutes
eyelids (both)	£500-£650
face lift	£600-£800
hair transplant	£7-12 per plug
nose surgery	£550-£750
squint correction	£400-£550
thigh and buttock lift	£650-£850

Glossary

Every effort has been made to avoid the use of medical jargon in the text. However, there are some terms used frequently by physicians and surgeons in reference to cosmetic surgery. Below is a list of such terms. The definitions are derived from *Dorland's Illustrated Medical Dictionary* (25th edition) and from *Blakiston's New Gould Medical Dictionary* (2nd edition). In cases in which the definitions were written in technical language, a physician or surgeon has translated them into terms understandable by a lay person.

abdominoplasty: surgery to remove hanging skin and/or stretch marks from the abdomen

acne: a chronic, inflammatory disease of the sebaceous glands, most often found on the face, chest, and back

adipose: fatty

ala: a winglike structure or process; in cosmetic surgery, the word most often refers to the flaring outer side of each nostril

alopecia: absence of the hair from skin areas where it is normally present

alopecia areata: an inflammatory, potentially reversible, loss of hair, usually involving the scalp

analgesic: an agent alleviating pain without causing loss of consciousness

anaesthesia: loss of sensation of pain, as it is induced to permit performance of surgery or other painful procedures

anaesthesia, general: a state of unconsciousness, produced by anaesthetic agents, with absence of pain sensation over the entire body. The drugs producing this state can be administered by inhalation, intravenously, intramuscularly, or via the gastrointestinal tract.

anaesthesia, local: anaesthesia confined to one part of the body

anterior: situated before or in front of

antihelix: the prominent semicircular ridge on the

221

external ear, just below the helix

antiseptic: preventing decay or putrefaction

areola: the darkened ring surrounding the nipple of the breast

asepis: freedom from infection

auricle; the portion of the external ear not contained within the head

axilla: the small hollow beneath the arm, where it joins the body at the shoulder

biopsy: the removal and examination, usually microscopic, of tissue from the living body for purposes of diagnosis

bite: relative position of the lower and upper teeth

blepharoplasty: plastic surgery of the eyelids

canthus: the corner on either side of the eyes where upper and lower lids meet

capillary: minute blood vessel

carcinogenic: producing cancer

carcinoma: a cancerous growth

cartilage: a fibrous, elastic connective tissue forming part of the skeleton

cervical: pertaining to the neck

chemosurgery: the destruction of skin by chemicals, producing an intense burn and then a peel

clavicle: the collarbone

coagulation: the process of clot formation

collagen: the main supportive protein of skin, tendon, bone, cartilage, and connective tissue

columella: the fleshy column below the tip of the nose

congenital: a condition present at birth

conjunctiva: the membrane that lines the eyelids and covers the exposed surface of the eyeball

cutaneous: pertaining to the skin

dermabrasion: mechanical abrading of the skin to remove the top layers

dermatitis: inflammation of the skin

dermatologist: a skin specialist

dermis: the layer of skin below the epidermis

dorsum: the back of a body part

dyscrasia: an abnormal condition of the blood

dysfunction: impairment or abnormality of the functioning of an organ

ectropion: a turning outwards, especially of an eyelid

epicanthus: a vertical fold of skin on either side of the nose

epidermis: the outer layer of the skin

excise: to cut out or off

fascia: a sheet or band of thick fibrous tissues that sheathes the muscles and various organs of the body

flap: a partially detached mass of skin and tissue with its own blood supply

frenulum: the fold of mucous membrane in the inside of the middle of the lips, connecting the lips with the gums

glabella: the area between the eyebrows

graft: tissue moved from one part of the body to another

haematoma: an abnormal collection of blood under the skin, caused by injury or surgery

haemostasis: the control of blood flow

helix: the rounded rim of the external ear

hyper-: a prefix signifying above, beyond, excessive

hypertrophy: enlargement or overgrowth

hypo-: a prefix signifying beneath, under, or deficient

hypotensive: causing low blood pressure or a lowering of blood pressure

implant: material inserted or grafted into the body

incision: a cut, or a wound produced by cutting

inferior: situated below, or directed downwards

keloid: an abnormal overgrowth of scar tissue

keratosis: a thickened, horny area of the skin

labial: pertaining to the lips

latissimas dorsi: muscle in the back used to pull the body up in climbing and as an accessory muscle of respiration

lipectomy: excision of fatty tissue

malocclusion: abnormal relationship between upper and lower teeth

mammaplasty: plastic reconstruction of the breast. Augmentation mammaplasty enlarges the breasts; reduction mammaplasty reduces the size

mandible: the bone of the lower jaw

mastectomy: excision of the breast
mastopexy: the surgical correction of a pendulous breast
maxilla: the upper jawbone
melanin: the dark pigment of the skin and hair
meloplasty: plastic surgery of the cheek
membrane: a thin layer of tissue which covers a surface,
    lines a cavity, or divides a space or organ
mentoplasty: plastic surgery of the chin
nasolabial fold: fold running from the side of the nose to
    the upper lip
necrosis: death of tissue
obesity: an excessive accumulation of fat in the body
occlusion: the relation of the upper and lower teeth
oedema: swelling produced by large amounts of fluid
oestrogen: female sex hormone
orbit: the bony cavity that contains the eyeball
osteotomy: the surgical cutting of a bone
octoplasty: plastic surgery of the ear
palpebral: pertaining to an eyelid
plaque: a patch or flat area
posterior: situated in back of, or in the back part of
preauricular: situated in front of the ear
prognathous: having projecting jaws
prosthesis: an artificial part
ptosis: drooping of the upper eyelid
rhinoplasty: plastic surgery of the nose
rhytidectomy: a face lift
sebum: an oily, waxlike substance secreted by the
    sebaceous glands
septum: a dividing wall or partition, as the nasal septum
slough: a mass of dead tissue cast out from living tissue
striae: stretch marks
subcutaneous: situated beneath the skin
submental: situated below the chin
suture: a stitch or series of stitches made to secure together
    the edges of a surgical or accidental wound
testosterone: the male hormone
transverse: placed horizontally
trichology: the study of the hair
umbilicus: the naval

vascular, vaso-: pertaining to the blood vessels
venous: pertaining to the veins
xanthoma: small flat plaques of yellow colour in the skin,
    often the eyelids
zygoma: the cheek bone